# Evaluating the Effectiveness of Voice Therapy
Second Edition

# Evaluating the Effectiveness of Voice Therapy

Functional, Organic and Neurogenic Voice Disorders

Second Edition

Paul Carding

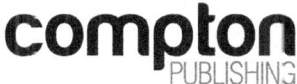

This edition first published 2017 © 2017 by Compton Publishing Ltd.
*Registered office:* Compton Publishing Ltd, 30 St. Giles', Oxford, OX1 3LE, UK
Registered company number: 07831037
*Editorial offices:* 35 East Street, Braunton, EX33 2EA, UK
Web: www.comptonpublishing.co.uk

The right of the authors to be identified as the authors of this work has been asserted in accordance with the UK Copyright, Designs and Patents Act 1988.

All rights reserved. No part of this publication may be reproduced, stored in a retrieval system, or transmitted, in any form or by any means, electronic, mechanical, photocopying, recording or otherwise, except as permitted by the UK Copyright, Designs and Patents Act 1988, without the prior permission of the publisher.

Trademarks: Designations used by companies to distinguish their products are often claimed as trademarks. Any brand names and product names used in this book are trade names, service marks, trademarks or registered trademarks of their respective owners. The publisher is not associated with any product or vendor mentioned in this book.

Disclaimer: This book is designed to provide helpful information on the subject discussed. This book is not meant to be used, nor should it be used, to diagnose or treat any medical condition. For diagnosis or treatment of any medical condition, consult your own physician. The publisher and author are not responsible for any specific medical condition that may require medical supervision and are not liable for any damages or negative consequences to any person reading or following the information in this book. References are provided for informational purposes only and do not constitute endorsement of any product, website, or other source.

Permissions: Where necessary, the publisher and author(s) have made every attempt to contact copyright owners and clear permissions for copyrighted materials. In the event that this has not been possible, the publisher invites the copyright owner to contact them so that the necessary acknowledgments can be made.

ISBN 978-1-909082-56-4

A catalogue record for this book is available from the British Library.

Cover image: Copyright Sebastian Kaulitzki. Courtesy of Shutterstock (www.shutterstock.com)

Cover design: David Siddall, http://www.davidsiddall.com

Set in 11pt Adobe Caslon by Regent Typesetting

# Contents

| | |
|---|---|
| List of contributing authors | vii |
| Foreword by Janet Wilson, FRCS(Ed), FRCS | 1 |
| Foreword by Robert E. Hillman, Ph.D | 1 |
| Foreword by Martin Birchall, FRCS | 1 |
| Introduction | 1 |
| 1. The need for evidence of treatment effectiveness<br>*Paul Carding* | 1 |
| 2. The importance of study design<br>*Paul Carding* | 7 |
| 3. The effectiveness of voice therapy for functional voice disorders<br>*Marianne Bos-Clark and Paul Carding* | 27 |
| 4. The effectiveness of voice therapy for vocal fold nodules<br>*Sherry Fu and Paul Carding* | 55 |
| 5. The effectiveness of voice therapy for mass lesions of the vocal folds<br>*Sue M. Jones and Paul Carding* | 81 |
| 6. The effectiveness of voice therapy for patients with unilateral vocal fold paralysis<br>*Chloe Walton and Paul Carding* | 99 |
| 7. The effectiveness of voice therapy for Parkinson's disease-related voice disorder<br>*Patricia Gillivan-Murphy and Paul Carding* | 113 |
| 8. Techniques for measuring voice outcomes of therapy interventions<br>*Paul Carding* | 135 |
| 9. The future<br>*Paul Carding* | 173 |
| Index | 183 |

# List of Contributing Authors

**Paul Carding Dip CCS., PhD., FRCSLT**

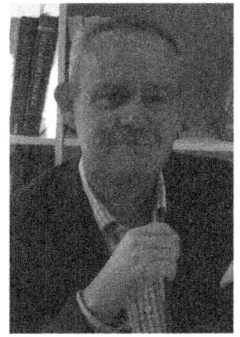

Professor Paul Carding has worked as an academic and clinical researcher for more than 25 years. He is currently Professor of Speech Pathology at Australian National Catholic University (Brisbane, Sydney and Melbourne). He also holds several other honorary positions including Senior Research Fellow at University College London (UK), Honorary Professor at Newcastle University (UK) and Visiting Professor at Strathclyde University (UK). Prof Carding has been awarded over $4 million in research grant funding and has published over 100 peer-reviewed articles as well as 15 book chapters and two books. He has supervised over 20 PhD and Masters students to completion and has been a keynote speaker at over 50 international conferences.

Prof Carding is a Fellow of the Royal College of Speech and Language Therapists (UK) and an honorary member of the Royal Society of Medicine (UK). He is also Speech Pathology national advisor to the Otolaryngology National Clinical Trials Office (UK). For over 20 years he was voice advisor to the Royal Shakespeare Company (UK). He is a regular reviewer of manuscripts for four international academic journals and has examined PhD students from a number of universities around the world.

**Marianne Bos-Clarke BSc., MSc., MRCSLT**

Marianne is the Lead Speech and Language Therapist for Voice and ENT at the Royal Devon and Exeter NHS Foundation Trust and a Lecturer at the University of St. Mark and St. John, Plymouth. In 2004, Marianne completed an MSc in Voice Disorders with distinction at Newcastle University. With over fifteen years of specialist experience in managing voice disorders, Marianne has taught widely, presented at conferences and published several articles. Research interests include Solution Focused Brief Therapy in voice therapy, the therapeutic application of the Estill model of voice and the effectiveness and content of voice therapy – particularly in functional dysphonia. Marianne is currently training to be a Certified Master Teacher of Estill.

### Sherry Fu BSc., PhD.
Dr Sherry Fu has been practicing as a bilingual speech-language pathologist for over 11 years in the fields of voice disorders, head and neck cancer and bilingual speech and language disorders. She is currently assistant professor of Department of Audiology and Speech Language Pathology at the Mackay Medical College (Taiwan) and part-time bilingual speech-language pathologist at Taipei American School (Taiwan). Dr Fu is also a supervisory board member of the Speech-Language-Hearing Association of Taiwan.

### Sue M Jones BSc., MSc., MRCSLT
Sue M. Jones has been working with Clinical Voice Disorders for 34 years. She co-directs the Voice Clinic Services at University Hospital of South Manchester, UK and heads a team of specialist voice therapists. Sue holds an MSc in Voice Research (Newcastle University) and is an adviser on Voice Disorders to the Royal College of Speech and Language Therapists as well as being the RCSLT representative for the British Laryngological Association. She has previously been a director of the British Voice Association. Sue published *Laryngeal Endoscopy and Voice Therapy: A Clinical Guide* (Compton Publishing) in 2016. She also specialises in the management of the injured professional singer and has worked in partnership with singing teachers and vocal coaches. Sue has led the development of a national training programme for perceptual analysis in the UK and presented extensively at major national and international meetings.

### Patricia Gillivan Murphy BSc., MSc, PhD
Patricia Gillivan-Murphy has over twenty five years clinical experience in voice disorders, with particular focus on clinical research over the past ten years. Currently, she works at the Mater Misericordiae University Hospital, Dublin as a Clinical Specialist (Voice).She carries a clinical caseload of patients with voice and swallowing disorders, teaches at an undergraduate and post graduate level and engages in clinical research. She is the clinical lead in Fiberoptic Endoscopic Evaluation of Swallowing (FEES) and teaches FEES locally and nationally. She achieved a Masters in clinical research (voice) in 2004 and a PhD in 2013 both from the University of Newcastle upon Tyne, UK. She has published research findings from studies on voice treatment effectiveness in teachers and voice tremor characteristics in Parkinson's disease.

**Chloe Walton BA., MSpPathSt**

Chloe Walton is a speech pathologist who completed her Master of Speech Pathology studies in 2009 at the University of Queensland, Australia. She has worked for several years within tertiary and private settings. During this time she has participated in a number of voice research projects. She has a particular clinical interest in the management of functional dysphonia and presented her findings at international forums including the Speech Pathology Australia National Conference in 2013. The resultant article entitled "Is more intensive better? Client and Service Provider Outcomes for Intensive versus standard therapy schedules for functional voice disorders" was published in the Journal of Voice. Chloe is currently a PhD student at Australian Catholic University where she is undertaking research into voice outcomes following surgical and behavioral management of patients with unilateral vocal fold paralysis.

# Dedication

The first edition of this book was dedicated to my family. It is a matter of enormous pride and comfort to me that this second edition is also dedicated to them.

Kate, my wife, remains a constant source of support and energy to me and I could not have written this book without her. James and Jeni are still my inspiration and I am hugely proud of them both.

# Acknowledgements

I am extremely grateful for the dedication and expertise of my co-authors. Thank you so much for your support and hard work.

A good decision is based on knowledge not on numbers.

Opinion is the medium between knowledge and ignorance.

Knowledge without justice ought to be called cunning rather than wisdom.

Plato (427–374 BCE)

# Foreword

It is a great pleasure to introduce this second edition of a unique and outstanding publication – *Evaluating the Effectiveness of Voice Therapy: Functional, Organic and Neurogenic Voice Disorders*. Professor Paul Carding is a leading proponent of evidence-based voice therapy worldwide and it is wonderful to watch his nurturing of a whole new generation of research-aware Speech and Language Therapists.

In any sphere of medicine, it is hard to establish a robust evidence base. No field is more challenging in this regard than that of client centred therapies, where the treatment choices are influenced by a wide range of patient and therapist factors and where controlling for variation in the delivery and acceptance of therapy interventions is equally problematic. Having first of all neatly summarised the core process of modern treatment evaluation, Paul and his team of highly specialised coauthors have done a marvellous job in assembling all the latest evidence sources in the published literature and presenting them in a lucid way, highly suited to the demands of busy clinicians seeking to review treatment options. The writing is uniformly scholarly, yet readable and the hard work of approaching a multi-layered topic has been done for the reader by the authors. While the general sections are invaluable to researchers and enquiring clinicians alike, the team has not shied away from the more demanding task of assessing the specific evidence for specific physical conditions, such as nodules, mass lesions and Parkinsonism.

This remarkable book serves several purposes. It presents evidence upon which treating therapists may formulate session plans with maximal cost efficacy, while pointing the way to evaluation of the relevant outcomes, in the context of what is already known. This volume therefore offers a comprehensive toolkit: literature appraisal; skills acquisition; highlights of key existing papers; and benchmarks against which to assess one's own practice.

This up to the minute volume is a most welcome addition to the published literature.

Janet A Wilson, B.Sc., MD, FRCS(Ed), FRCS(Eng), FRCSLT(Hon)
Professor, Otolaryngology and Head and Neck Surgery
Newcastle University, UK

# Foreword

In *Evaluating the Effectiveness of Voice Therapy: Functional, Organic and Neurogenic Voice Disorders*, Professor Carding has created an invaluable resource for students, clinicians and researchers interested in the behavioral management of common voice disorders. It provides an extremely logical and coherent approach to this topic by first establishing a solid foundation in the basic concepts related to gathering and assessing the quality of scientific evidence for treatment efficacy and effectiveness. Subsequent chapters are then devoted to cogent reviews of the evidence that currently exists for the effectiveness of voice therapy in treating specific types of voice disorders, as well the state-of-the art in voice outcome measures. The book concludes with a very balanced summary of the current evidence for voice therapy effectiveness, with practical suggestions about the types of future research that is needed to continue to build the evidence base.

For students in training to be voice clinicians, *Evaluating the Effectiveness of Voice Therapy: Functional, Organic and Neurogenic Voice Disorders* provides a wealth of clearly presented information about the current state of the evidence for voice therapy effectiveness; it also demonstrates the type of clinical reasoning that is critical for students to learn so that they can continue to interpret and apply new research findings as independent clinicians. For practicing clinicians, it can help facilitate informed treatment decisions and provide the information needed to explain the scientific bases for such decisions to colleagues, patients and their families. Finally, for researchers, this book literally provides a roadmap for pursuing the types of research that is needed to advance clinical practice in the behavioral management of voice disorders.

Robert E. Hillman, Ph.D.
Massachusetts General Hospital
Harvard Medical School
Boston, USA

# Foreword

Electronic communication reaches deep into society, work and the eyes, minds and hands of children. However, these typed words fail to convey context, social and emotional import and, ultimately deeper layers of meanings. It appears that true depth communication requires the human voice. Voice remains the most powerful, effective and, therefore, most used communication medium of our age and therefore the protection and restoration of vocal health is one of the greatest responsibilities of healthcare and health research.

This book is a beacon lit to signal the need to scale-up research efforts into voice disorders. It is also a light to attract those seeking a way to advance the field for benefit of both patients and voice science per se. With all health care coming under global scrutiny, this signal could not be more timely. Professor Carding set out his stall here by putting the importance and design of voice research upfront, for all that follows in terms of describing disorders and their care depends entirely on evidence. Voice therapy has come of age and this book, as well as clearly laying out ways of treatment and research, is a wonderful celebration of this moment in time. I know both serious and casual readers will quickly join the party.

Martin Birchall, FRCS
Professor of Laryngology, Consultant Laryngologist and Head and Neck Surgeon and NIHR Senior Investigator
University College London

# Introduction

The first edition of the book entitled *Evaluating Voice Therapy: Measuring the Effectiveness of Treatment* was published early in 2000. A number of significant developments have happened in the field of voice disorders since that time. For example, in 2000, The Voice Handicap Index (Jacobson et al., 1997) had only just started to be used and other significant patient reports such as the Voice Activation and Participation Profile (Ma and Yiu, 2001) and The Voice Symptom Scale (Deary et al., 2003) had not been published. Similarly, the pivotal evidence for intensive voice treatment for patients with Parkinson's disease (Ramig et al., 2001) was not to be published until October 2001. The first Cochrane systematic review of voice therapy for any type of voice disorder did not happen until 2007 (Ruotsalainen et al., 2007). In fact, arguably, the whole evidence-based practice movement had hardly begun to gather impetus – Sackett's seminal book on how to practice and teach evidence-based medicine (Sackett et al., 1998) was not published in 1998. Greenhalgh's equally influential book on how to read a research paper (Greenhalgh, 2001) did not follow until 2001. And since the first edition of this book there have been a large number of new and important studies of voice therapy effectiveness for many different types of voice disorder. Ironically, the number of studies probably means that the busy voice clinician is unlikely to be unable to keep up. One of the purposes of this book is therefore to provide the voice clinician with all of the relevant speech pathology intervention effectiveness evidence for a range of different voice disorders

This second edition, entitled *Measuring the Effectiveness of Voice Therapy: Functional, Organic and Neurogenic Voice Disorders*, provides a summary and critical appraisal of all of the relevant speech pathology treatment effectiveness studies published between 2005 and 2015. As the title suggests, this represents an evaluation of the literature across the three main etiological groups of voice disorders that readily utilise speech pathology as a primary and/or adjunct treatment modality. Similar to the first edition, the book contains several preliminary chapters on the importance of study design and techniques for measuring voice outcomes over time. However, these chapters have been significantly re-written. This is followed by a series of chapters that critically evaluate the effectiveness of voice therapy in Functional Voice Disorders (Chapter 3), Vocal Nodules (Chapter 4), Organic Voice Disorders (Chapter 5), Unilateral Vocal Fold Paralysis (Chapter 6) and Neurological Voice Disorders: Parkinson's Disease (Chapter 7). I am hugely grateful to my co-authors for their devotion and commitment to writing these chapters. The final chapter allows for a look into the future and asks whether we have enough high quality studies, how do we apply the findings to individuals in our practice and how do we embark on the next phases of the dissemination of our evidence base.

## References

Deary IJ, Wilson JA, Carding PN *et al.* (2003) VoiSS: a patient derived voice symptom scale. *Journal of Psychosomatic Research* **54**: 483–489

Greenhalgh T. (2001) *How to Read a Paper: The Basics of Evidence Based Medicine* London: BMJ Books.

Jacobson BH, Johnson A, Grywalski S *et al.* (1997) The Voice Handicap Index; development and validation *American Journal of Speech and Language Pathology* **6**: 66–70. doi 1044/1058-0360.0603.66

Ma E, Yiu E (2001) Voice activity and participation profile: assessing the impact of voice disorders on daily activities *Journal of Speech and Hearing Research* **44**: 511–24

Ramig L, Sapir S, Countryman S *et al.* (2001) Intensive voice treatment (LSVT®) for patients with Parkinson's disease: a 2 year follow up *Journal of Neurology, Neurosurgery and Psychiatry* **71**: 493–98.

Ruotsalainen, JH. Sellman, J. Lehto, L *et al.* (2007) Interventions for treating functional dysphonia in adults *The Cochrane Library* **3**:1–29.

Sackett D, Richardson W, Rosenberg W, Haynes RB (1998) *Evidence Based Medicine: How to Practice and Teach EBM* London: Churchill Livingstone.

# The need for evidence of treatment effectiveness

## Paul Carding

### Why do we still need evidence of treatment effectiveness?

All people involved in health care have the same goal: to provide the most effective care available and to achieve the best outcome for the patient. Evidence of treatment effectiveness is central for (a) patient care, (b) professional integrity, (c) service provision and (d) clinical research. It is important to explain these concepts further.

### Patient care

Evaluating the evidence of treatment effectiveness allows clinicians to provide patients with the best treatment possible. It allows for the delivery of the intervention most likely to improve the patient's outcome for a given clinical condition. Patients have every right to think that they are being offered the most up-to-date and efficacious (and efficient) intervention, given their presenting condition and individual circumstances. Evidence of the efficacy of treatment is necessary to "offer an improved quality of life … as effectively as possible to the maximum number of people" (Enderby, 1995). Patient expectation has become more focused with increased ability to access information from the internet.

## Professional integrity

Clinicians have a professional obligation to provide the "best" treatment for the individual patient. The treating clinician needs to access the evidence, assess the accuracy of this information, determine the suitability of the evidence for the individual client and discuss whether this intervention is the most appropriate and effective option. It is therefore incumbent upon the practising clinician to be up-to-date with the evidence (or at least able to access this information) and be sufficiently skilled to deliver the treatment that is indicated, as described by Hoffman *et al.* (2013):

> *"When we integrate the best available evidence with information from our clinical knowledge, patients and practice context, the reasoning behind our clinical decisions becomes more apparent and this serves to reinforce both our professional accountability and our claim of being a health professional" (page 6).*

## Service provision

Governments, policy-makers and service providers are inevitably concerned with health expenditure. The allocation of limited financial resources is based (although not exclusively) on information about the efficacy and effectiveness of current interventions. They wish to maximise the provision of health resources to the largest population possible.

> *"The competitive edge will go to the health care professionals who can demonstrate most effectively – based on hard data what beneficial outcomes their services can deliver" (Boston, 1994).*

## Clinical research

Many specialist areas of speech pathology have developed from an anecdotal base and some still lack an academic, or even theoretical, underpinning (Reilly *et al.*, 2004). Whilst this is no longer the case in many areas of voice therapy, there are still many questions about clinical practice that remain unanswered. Collation and critical appraisal of the evidence of effectiveness of intervention, highlights areas of strength but also areas of research weakness. Some areas of voice therapy only have a small and poor quality evidence base and this requires significant research investment to provide valuable data to support (and change) clinical practice. Other areas of voice therapy have a well established evidence base, although here too important clinical questions have yet to be answered. These will be highlighted in the subsequent chapters of this book

## The concept of evidence-based practice

Clearly linked to this pursuit of evidence of treatment effectiveness is the concept of evidence-based practice (EBP). The critical evaluation and dissemination of treatment effectiveness is a key aspect of EBP but not the only one. For example, EBP is also concerned with diagnostic effectiveness. The definition of EBP has been refined over time. It is now commonly considered to be the integration of the best research evidence with clinical expertise and the patient's own unique values and circumstances (Hoffman et al., 2013). This is perhaps more holistic than the original definition of evidence-based medicine provided by Sackett and colleagues (Sackett et al., 1998): "Evidence-based medicine is the conscientious, explicit and judicious use of current best evidence in making decisions about the care of individual patients" (page 2). Evidence-based healthcare has also been described as "a discipline centred upon evidence-based decision-making about groups of patients, or populations, which may be manifest as evidence-based policy-making, purchasing or management (Gray, 1997).The key to all of these definitions is that EBP is considered a way of implementing practice that involves an individualised, thoughtful process of using the evidence to make the best decisions for any given patient.

Greenhalgh (2001) reminds us that the main enemy of EBP is expert opinion. Whilst expert opinion can of course be a highly valuable source of information, it is not strictly evidence at all unless it can be supported by high quality scientific data. Expert opinion can be very biased and it is perhaps more common than we care to admit. This is "eminence-based" rather the "evidence-based" practice. Equally misleading is pseudo-expert opinion. For example, modern media outlets may enable (and even encourage) irresponsible reporting of "evidence" which may be "believed" by the undiscerning reader. It is incumbent upon any professional to judge the quality of the evidence via critical appraisal and certainly not to rely on the reports of potentially biased and/or unqualified journalists.

## Levels of evidence

Not all sources of published evidence are equal. Clinicians and researchers (as well as the public) are required to differentiate strong from weak evidence. It is common to refer to hierarchies of evidence which provide a ranking according to the relative value from high to low. It is a useful means of identifying study types of varying levels of methodological trustworthiness (i.e., free from bias). In general, studies that are higher in the hierarchy represent more robust methodology and hence produce results of efficacy which are scientifically strong and more likely to be trustworthy. A low level or weak study implies that there has been no or little scientific evaluation, or that the methodology used limits the trustworthiness or generalisability of the results. These matters of methodological design are the subject of Chapter 2. Table 1 is a simplified version of a hierarchy of evidence developed by the National Health and Medical Research Council of Australia (1999).

Table 1: Hierarchies and Levels of Evidence for Intervention Effectiveness

| Level | Study design |
| --- | --- |
| I | A systematic review of Level II studies |
| II | Randomised controlled trial |
| III-1 | Pseudo-randomised controlled trial |
| III-2 | Comparative study with concurrent controls<br>• non-randomised<br>• experimental trial<br>• cohort study<br>• case-control study<br>• interrupted time-series with control group |
| III-3 | Comparative study *without* concurrent controls<br>• historical control study<br>• two or more single arm study<br>• interrupted time-series without a parallel control group |
| IV | Case series<br>Case studies |

It is however important to note that it would be misleading to think that a poorly designed or implemented randomised controlled study is superior to a well designed controlled group study (for example). The ranking of evidence in a hierarchy is not a substitute for accurate critical appraisal. Equally, as discussed in Chapter 2, some areas of clinical practice are in their relative infancy and hence, in these areas, Level IV case studies and series are highly appropriate. Finally, it is important to note that Level I evidence in the Table below does not represent an efficacy study with data at all. Rather it is a collation of the evidence from previously published Level II studies. Again, this will be explained in detail in Chapter 2.

It has been argued that the hierarchy listed in Table 1 is quite difficult to understand and refers to a number of study designs which rarely occur in behavioural sciences such as voice therapy practice. Many authors prefer to use the levels of evidence from the Joanna Briggs Institute for Evidence-based Nursing and Midwifery for the evaluation of treatment (www.joannabriggs.edu.au). The levels of evidence appear to be less complicated and clearly applicable to behavioural interventions. This hierarchy also includes different Level IV evidence which acknowledges opinion of respected authorities, clinical experience and reports of expert committees. Strictly speaking this is not evidence at all but has been adopted in some areas of speech pathology where there is an absence of any other information of intervention effectiveness. Fortunately, for the evaluation of voice therapy effectiveness, this Level IV is not required (and not reported on in this book). Nevertheless, for the purposes of completeness, the Joanna Briggs levels of evidence are presented in Table 2 below.

Table 2: The Joanna Briggs Institute Levels of Evidence for Intervention Effectiveness

| Level | |
|---|---|
| I | Evidence obtained from a systematic review of all relevant randomised controlled trials |
| II | Evidence obtained from at least one properly designed randomised controlled trial |
| III-1 | Evidence obtained from well-designed controlled trials without randomisation |
| III-2 | Evidenced obtained from well-designed cohort or case control analytic studies, preferably from more than one centre or research group |
| III-3 | Evidence obtained from multiple time series, with or without the intervention<br>Dramatic results in uncontrolled experiments |
| IV | Opinion of respected authorities, based on clinical experience, descriptive studies or reports of expert committees |

Based on Joanna Briggs Institute for Evidence-based Nursing and Midwifery (www.joannabriggs.edu.au)

## The structure of this book

The next chapter addresses the importance of study design in determining the effectiveness of treatment. This includes a description of the more common designs used, as well as details concerning study validity and statistical concepts. The following five chapters address the literature and evidence base for particular types of voice disorders: Functional Voice Disorders (Chapter 3), Vocal Nodules (Chapter 4), Organic Voice Disorders (Chapter 5), Unilateral Vocal Fold Paralysis (Chapter 6) and Parkinson's Disease Voice Disorder (Chapter 7). Each of these chapters includes a summary table of all relevant voice treatment efficacy and effectiveness studies. Chapter 8 is concerned with voice outcome measurement; first, it describes the importance of choosing the most appropriate measure before summarising the most common voice outcome measures used in the literature. A summary table of studies that have used each of the more common outcome measures is provided. The final chapter includes a summary of the state of the evidence base for the speech pathology treatment of voice disorders and a consideration of the priorities for future research in this field of expertise.

## References

Boston BO (1994) Destiny is in the data: A wake-up call for outcome measures. *ASHA Leader* 36(11):35-38.

Enderby P and Emmerson J (1995) *Does Speech and Language Therapy Work?* London: Whurr Publishers.

Gray JAM (1997) *Evidence-based Healthcare* (2edn) New York, NY: Churchill Livingstone.

Greenhalgh T (2001) *How to Read a Paper: The Basics of Evidence Based Medicine* London: BMJ Books.

Hoffman T, Bennett A and del Mar C (2013) *Evidence-based Practice Across the Health Professions* (2edn). New York, NY: Church Livingstone Elsevier.

National Health and Medical Research Council (NHMRC) (1999) *How to review the evidence: Systematic identification and review of scientific literature.* 1999; Available from: http://www.nhmrc.gov.au/_files_nhmrc/publications/attachments/cp65.pdf [Accessed August 2016].

Reilly S, Douglas J and Oates J (2004) *Evidence-based Practice in Speech Pathology.* London: Whurr Publishers.

Sackett D, Richardson W, Rosenberg W, Haynes RB (1998) *Evidence-based Medicine: How to Practice and Teach EBM.* London: Churchill Livingstone.

# 2

# The importance of study design

## Paul Carding

The nature and quality of the study design is crucial when considering the treatment effectiveness evidence base in any given field. The assessment of the evidence is essentially a process of determining how "believable" and relevant the study is/studies are. Key to this assessment is the identification of the types of study that have been used to measure the relationship between treatment and outcome. There may be many reasons why a patient has improved and it may be misleading to assume that because the improvement results from the treatment given. The quality of evidence is essentially a hierarchy of study design which is more likely to prove that the change in a patient's performance is a direct result of the treatment rather than from spontaneous improvement or from other (non-controlled) interacting factors. To be confident of the cause and effect relationship between treatment and outcome we need to be as convinced as possible (we can never be absolutely sure) that there has been appropriate control of independent and dependent variables and accurate data interpretation.

There are three fundamental reasons why we might not believe the evidence presented from a particular study. These are as follows:

(1) *Using the wrong type of study design for the question*
    The study used the wrong design to answer the specific research question. There are many study designs available (see section below) and that is because "no size fits all". Using the wrong study design will result in no direct answer to the research question or a biased answer to the question.

(2) *Flaws in the conduct of the study*

Even when the research design is appropriate for the research question, poor study conduct can contaminate the results to such an extent that they are of limited value. Examples of poor study conduct include: poor attention to inclusion/exclusion criteria, inaccurate measurement, unwanted variance between key variables such as the treatment given, treatment duration, re-assessment timings, inaccurate analysis and inadequate documentation for replication purposes. If a study is inadequate in a number of important ways the reader may be unsure whether the apparent "results" are believable and trustworthy.

(3) *Insufficient numbers of study participants*

Many studies are "under powered" for finding a meaningful difference between one group and another, or between one treatment and another. It seems obvious that the effectiveness of treatment may not be shown to be significant in a study of, say, 10 people, but may represent a real difference that can only be shown with larger numbers of patients. It is important that effectiveness studies are sufficiently "powered" to determine a real difference. This concept of statistical power is explained later in this chapter.

## Explaining different study types

Chapter 1 includes a table of the hierarchies and levels of evidence for intervention effectiveness. It is reproduced again here. These hierarchies explain the type of studies that provide the most robust (the least likelihood of bias) evidence. It is important to explain this further with a brief explanation of what these types of study design are and how they work.

Table 1: Hierarchies and Levels of Evidence for Intervention Effectiveness

| Level | Study design |
|---|---|
| I | A systematic review of Level II studies |
| II | Randomised controlled trial |
| III-1 | Pseudo-randomised controlled trial |
| III-2 | Comparative study with concurrent controls<br>• non-randomised<br>• experimental trial<br>• cohort study<br>• case-control study<br>• interrupted time-series with control group |
| III-3 | Comparative study without concurrent controls<br>• historical control study<br>• two or more single arm studies<br>• interrupted time-series without a parallel control group |
| IV | Case series<br>Case studies |

## Systematic reviews

Systematic reviews are a means of synthesising the literature on a particular topic. There are a number of systematic reviews in the voice literature which are described in detail in the relevant chapters of this book. Systematic reviews are different from literature reviews in that they follow a transparent, explicit and pre-defined methodology which is designed to limit bias. Systematic reviews are intended to be comprehensive and trustworthy methods of capturing and synthesising the literature. Cook *et al.* (1997) state that the main differences of literature reviews as opposed to systematic reviews are as follows:

a. They employ clear eligibility and inclusion criteria
b. They incorporate a comprehensive and transparent search strategy to identify all potentially relevant studies (including those published in all languages)
c. They are explicit about the criteria applied in the selection of studies in the review and ensure that this methodology is reproducible and applied consistently across all potential studies
d. They explicitly appraise the risk of bias in all studies that are included in the review
e. They systematically synthesise the results of included studies.

With a number of quantitative studies (n = 2+) results are typically summarised using a measure of effect size and meta-analysis (a means of combining results from multiple studies).

Hoffmann *et al.* (2013) explain the basic steps of conducting a systematic review:

a. Define the research question and plan the methods for undertaking the review
b. Determine the eligibility criteria for studies to be included
c. Search for potential eligible studies
d. Apply eligibility criteria to select studies
e. Assess the risk of bias in included studies
f. Extract data from the included studies
g. Interpret and report the results.

## A randomised controlled trial (RCT)

RCTs are considered the best type of study to determine the effectiveness of an intervention or the comparative effectiveness of one intervention over another. Participants are randomised into two (or more) different groups in order to randomly distribute variables which may otherwise influence treatment outcome. There is, in addition, control of the major independent variables (for example, subject/participant characteristics and the details of the treatment programme). The participants in the two (or more) groups receive a different intervention (one of which may be a 'no-treatment' group). At the end of the trial, the effects of the different interventions are measured. Whilst this study design is universally regarded as the most robust, there is also an acknowledgment that it is (a) very difficult to achieve in many areas of behavioural intervention and (b) not always the most appropriate design for all treatment effectiveness research questions.

## A pseudo-randomised controlled trial

This type of study is similar to a randomised controlled trial but, as the name suggests, it uses a different ("not-quite-randomised") client/patient allocation procedure. The allocation of participants is carried out using a selection process (e.g., matching of participants according to sex, age or other criteria) or allocation by date of birth, hospital record number or alternation.

## Comparative study design with concurrent controls

- *Non-randomised experimental trial*
  As the name suggests, this is essentially the same as a randomised controlled study except that the subjects are not randomly allocated to the different treatment groups. Participants are allocated to treatment and no-treatment (control) groups by other means (for example, sequential allocation) and the outcomes from each group are compared. The lack of randomisation obviously opens the possibility of biased allocation in the groups. A lot of trials based in clinical facilities fall into this category because true randomisation may not be possible for a number of practical and logistical reasons.

- *Cohort study*
  A cohort refers to a group of participants with specific (identified) characteristics. Cohort studies typically follow these participants over time and differences are measured between them and in comparison with a controlled cohort.

- *Case-control study*
  Individual cases who receive an intervention are compared with individual cases who do not receive the intervention but who are "matched" to the treated cases. This matching is used to 'cancel out' the important other variables. For example, cases can be matched for age, sex, stage of disease, severity and/or length since onset.

- *Interrupted time-series with control group*
  This design measures outcomes (e.g., from treatment) at multiple points in time. These measures should occur both before and after treatment. The results are compared with a group of subjects who did not receive the treatment but were measured at the same time-points. One application of this design is to measure long-term effects of treatment and/or to measure the cumulative effect of a prolonged treatment programme.

## Comparative study without concurrent controls

- *Historical control study*
  As the name suggests, the control group in this type of study is not concurrent with the experimental/intervention group. The data from the prospective group who receive the intervention of interest are compared with either (a) data from a previously published study or (b) previous data collected from the same institution before the introduction of the intervention of interest: a control group who have received "standard" care. The use of historical control data is only valid if the patient group and outcome measures are sufficiently similar in the group who receive the intervention of interest.

- *Two or more single arm studies*
  This is a study design that uses the data collected from two or more studies both of which have a single series of participants. Although these studies are usually independent from one another, the participants will have received the same treatment of interest. Clearly, this design is only feasible if the participants in each study are comparable (e.g., similar inclusion /exclusion criteria) and the outcomes that are measured are the same.

- *Interrupted time-series without a parallel control group*
  This is the same study design as that described above but without a control group. Hence, this study design is seen as "weaker" and less scientifically robust.

## Case series/case studies

This design is simply a description of a series of patients/clients who have been given the intervention being evaluated. Clearly, the rationale here is that the more case studies reported, the larger the case series becomes and therefore, the more convincing are the effects of treatment. Case studies and case series are commonly used to describe a "proof of concept" and are an excellent means of describing a new or emerging treatment concept which may need refining or replicating a number of times before it can be established as worthy of further investigation. Case series are therefore able to produce interesting early results which may lead to a more definitive hypothesis testing and the consequent employment of more robust study designs.

## The five-phase model of efficacy/effectiveness research

Robey (2004) argues that evaluation of treatment effectiveness must also be considered within a broader organising structure for conducting clinical-outcome research activities. His five-phase model (Table 2 below) describes a logically ordered sequence from initial 'proof of concept' through various stages of "treatment efficacy" and then "treatment effectiveness" through to complete adaptation into clinical practice. Treatment efficacy research (Phase 1–3) examines clinical outcomes in an environment that "minimises all sources of extraneous or confounding variation" and "indexes the maximum potential of a treatment protocol for bringing about change" (page 402). In contrast, treatment effectiveness research examines the benefit of an intervention "provided in a typical fashion by typical practitioners to typical patients in typical clinical settings" (page 402). Therefore, the ultimate goal is evidence of treatment effectiveness, but effectiveness can only be tested when efficacy has been firmly established. However, as Pring (2005) highlights, these essential phases of building an evidence base can often be overlooked in the "rush" to publish large group trials and make claims about clinical effectiveness.

The five levels are summarised in Table 2 below.

While there still remains some debate, there is a reasonable argument that many areas of voice therapy treatment effectiveness have historically progressed through Phases 1 and 2 and are now situated in Phases 3 and 4. This is certainly the over-riding impression from many of the specific chapters of treatment effectiveness in this book. New interventions should of course begin again at Phase 1. However, as Pring (2005) highlights, these essential phases of building an evidence base can often be overlooked in the "rush" to publish large group trials.

## Table 2: The Five-phase Model of Clinical Outcomes Research

| Phase | Description |
|---|---|
| Phase 1 | • Aiming to detect the presence of a therapeutic effect by using single case studies, small-group pre-post studies and retrospective studies<br>• Research that explores and specifies the therapeutic effect as the main dependent variable<br>• Detection of an effect would provide justification of further investigation. |
| Phase 2 | • Aiming to refine the population to be studied, define the treatment protocol and determine the most appropriate assessments<br>• This is likely to involve deciding selection (inclusion/exclusion) criteria, defining duration and delivery of treatment and selecting/developing outcome measures<br>• Likely to include case-control series, small-group within effect studies and small-group (experimental vs control) studies<br>• Establishing the validity and reliability of measurement instruments (where this does not already exist)<br>• Making the necessary preparations for conducting a clinical trial. |
| Phase 3 | • Testing treatment efficacy using larger scale studies (a clinical trial to test efficacy)<br>• These designs will usually use a control group or a "treatment as normal" control group<br>• The results of a well-designed and documented study should be confirmed by independent replications<br>• Concerned with internal study validity. |
| Phase 4 | • Using large-scale effectiveness studies to determine whether the treatment effects observed in efficacy studies also translate into a clinical environment<br>• Aiming, where possible, to expand the applicability of the treatment protocol beyond stringent methodological conditions<br>• Refinement (expansion or reduction) of patient selection criteria<br>• Variations in treatment delivery, dosage and additional outcome measures<br>• Concerned with external study validity. |
| Phase 5 | • Aiming to determine the cost-effectiveness of the treatment and to assess consumer satisfaction and broader issues pertaining to the social and political environment of health service delivery<br>• Costs and values are assessed in fiscal terms through cost-effectiveness studies<br>• Costs and values are assessed in societal terms through cost–benefit analysis. |

## Common flaws in study design

Despite the obvious importance of observing the hierarchical structure of high quality and robust study design, it is important to note that a well-designed case series can be more meaningful than a poorly designed (or not quite relevant) randomised controlled study. Rosenfeld (1995) describes a number of common flaws in study design which should alert us from simply assuming that a study title or study design category will guarantee that the study has been well conducted. Needless to say authors may go some way to try to 'hide' the imperfections in their published works and so the reader may have difficulty in identifying them. This is a fundamental skill of critical appraisal. Some common design flaws are described below and some of them are illustrated in the literature reviews that follow in the subsequent chapters.

### Hypothetical hypotheses

These are studies that do not have a clear purpose. The study goal and/or hypothesis should be clearly and succinctly articulated. In many cases, this is clearly placed as the concluding statement at the end of the literature review. Equally common is when the study hypothesis is formulated *after* the collection of the data and yet written as though it was formulated at the onset. Obviously this is easier to identify if the study hypothesis/goals do not appear until the discussion section of the manuscript.

### Schizophrenic study type

These are studies that are labelled as one type of study design but which are, in fact, mislabelled. Perhaps more commonly, they "start out" by attempting to be one study design but, in reality, they are something different. For example, some review articles are presented as though they were prospective studies, or, as another example, a case series may be written as though it was a prospective group study. Rosenfeld (1995) states that most retrospective studies are commonly case series and most prospective studies appear as (but are not) randomised controlled studies. In both of these examples of course, the "level" of evidence is "lower" than the authors would wish the reader to believe.

## Unrepresentative samples

These are studies which use a sample of patients that do not reflect the clinical population in question. For example, the patients used in a given study may be younger, older, less complex, more motivated, more educated etc. than the general clinical population. In these cases it is not possible to generalise the results beyond the study sample itself. This is a criticism that is commonly held against studies that have applied very strict inclusion and exclusion criteria – where the resultant study sample is unlike any "real life" clinical population. Generalisation of a study's results can only occur if the study sample is representative of the intended clinical population.

## Clandestine controls

These studies create a control group where one didn't really exist! Most commonly they create a control group retrospectively (e.g., after the data has been collected for the treatment group) or fortuitously (e.g., collecting data on a group of patients who have not had the treatment that is being evaluated). There is major potential for bias (intended or unintended) in this practice. Less common is the use of historical controls (from previous studies or from other researchers). This is only justifiable if the two studies are identical and the time scale between them is not relevant.

## Confounded outcomes

The issue of confounding variables is discussed in the section below. "Confounding" refers to an apparent association between two variables where no association really exists. With respect to confounding *outcomes* in particular, this refers to the misappropriation of the relationship between an outcome and a treatment. It may be misleading to conclude that the outcome was the result of an intervention given. There may, of course, be many reasons why an outcome has changed (improved), including maturation, spontaneous recovery, change in other life circumstances and a change in (unreported) medications. This misinterpretation is most commonly seen in the discussion of statistical correlations between variables. Correlation does not mean causation; a correlation may or may not mean that the two variables are related in some way.

# Independent and dependent variables

## Independent variables

The heart of study design is concerned with the manipulation of the independent variable(s). In an efficacy or effectiveness study, these independent variables are those conditions that are carefully manipulated by the researcher to produce change. It gives the researcher the opportunity to measure the effects of the variables without the contamination of other major factors which may influence treatment outcome. If a major variable (i.e., one that is likely to influence treatment outcome) is not manipulated, then it should be controlled (Carding, 2000). In efficacy research, the major independent variables are subject/patient characteristics and the details of the treatment programme. Generally speaking, in the voice therapy literature, researchers have attempted to *control* the subject/patient characteristics and *manipulate* the treatment variable.

Control of subject/patient characteristics is most commonly achieved by specifying inclusion and exclusion criteria for participants in the study. This ensures that all patients share certain characteristics (e.g., non-smokers, no previous voice therapy, no previous history of voice problems, the same laryngeal diagnosis). This assumes that these are likely to be the most important individual characteristics (although this may not have been fully established). Other independent subject variables, such as educational background, patient motivation, severity of disorder etc., may or may not also be controlled if the researcher considers them to pose a sufficient risk to the integrity of the treatment outcome data. Of course, they can be manipulated while the treatment programme remains constant in order to observe the change in outcome. In this situation these manipulated variables are the core substance and purpose of the study.

However, understandably, treatment efficacy research mostly involves manipulating the treatment variable. These manipulations can take many forms. It would appear that most efficacy studies manipulate the *strength* and/or the *integrity* of the treatment programme. Strength refers to the frequency or intensity of treatment. Integrity refers to the details of the treatment programme (e.g., the components and stages of a treatment programme). This is the most common manipulation of the independent variables that we will see in the following chapters.

It is neither possible nor desirable to control every independent variable. By definition, less important independent variables should have a minimal impact on the outcomes of the study. Random allocation of participants assumes that the effects of these less important variables will dissipate across the treatment groups. Over control of minor independent variables will condemn a study to appearing not to reflect clinical practice and threaten its external validity (see section below).

## Dependent variables

In treatment efficacy/effectiveness studies, the dependent variables are the outcome measures. These dependent variables must include measures that provide data which assesses the nature and magnitude of the observed change. In voice disorders research this is not a simple matter. Voice is a complex multi-factorial phenomenon (Carding, 2000) and no one "voice measure" will encompass all of the important aspects that may change as a consequence of treatment. This matter is discussed in more detail in Chapter 8. The choice of outcome measures should be clearly related to the specific nature of the research question. If treatment is aimed at increasing vocal volume (loudness) then specific outcome measures can be used (for example, a sound pressure level meter). Similarly, if the goal of treatment is to enable the patient to use their voice successfully in their daily life then measuring vocal handicap and vocal participation can be used. However, in most voice therapy treatment efficacy/effectiveness studies, a number of outcome measures are employed (because any one measure is too specific and limited). However, many studies may select a 'primary' outcome measure and a series of "secondary" outcome measures. The primary outcome measure is usually the outcome tool that has been used in order to perform the *a priori* power calculation (see below).

Chapter 8 includes a discussion about the continuing debate over the relative merits of quantitative and qualitative outcomes data. Quantitative data refer to numerical data; observable, countable and quantifiable (usually on an equal interval appearing scale). The attractiveness of these data is still present in the current literature because (a) they may be seen as more "objective" and less "subjective" and (b) they are data that are conducive to statistical analysis. Qualitative data are descriptive, observational and interpretative. Traditional voice measures, such as perceptual voice quality judgement and laryngeal examination, provide qualitative, descriptive data. However, there are many tools that now "convert" these observations and interpretations into numerical (severity) data. The "subjectivity" of these measures is usually addressed by careful study design (for example employing "blind" raters with calculations of inter- and intra-rater reliability). Hence, most recent voice therapy effectiveness studies use a suite of outcome measures to reflect the complexity of the human voice.

## Internal validity of a study

The internal validity of a study essentially refers to how "believable" it is. The whole purpose of critical evaluation of the literature is to apply fundamental scientific design principles to determine whether the results are worthy of valued consideration and possible adoption into our clinical practice. The reader needs to know whether the results from a study are "trustworthy", and that they are not in truth due to some other factor. An apparent treatment effect or association may be untrustworthy if the study design and data analysis have not taken into account other factors that may impact treatment outcome. Fundamentally, these other factors are: (1) the impact of chance, (2) the impact of bias and (3) the impact of confounding variables. These are explained further below.

## Chance

One possible explanation for a study's results is that findings of differences between two groups are simply due to random variation or chance. However well a treatment study is designed, there is a chance that the difference between the groups is simply because one group just happens to contain more participants who responded positively. Any difference can occur by chance and there is always the possibility (or the level of probability) that this is due to random variation between subjects in the study. Determining whether findings are due to chance is a key feature of statistical analysis. Statistical tests calculate the probability of a chance result. If the probability is small we say that it is "statistically significant" and we are reasonably confident that the differences observed between the groups are *not* due to chance. If the probability is large, then the differences will not be statistically significant and we are not at all confident that they are due to the treatment under investigation.

## Bias

In contrast to chance, bias refers to systematic error in one or various aspects of a study design. These areas of bias may or may not be intentional on the part of the study designers. Bias can most commonly occur when recruiting participants for a study, during the measurement of the outcome results, or during the analysis of the data. Any or all of these aspects of bias will lead to, at best, inaccurate results and, at worst, misleading and plainly erroneous results.

Hoffman *et al.* (2010) provide a valuable synopsis of some of the more common types of study bias seen in treatment effectiveness studies. These are as follows:

- *Selection or sampling bias* occurs when there are systematic differences between those who are selected for the study and those who are not selected. This restricts the relevance or "generalisability" of the study findings to the general clinical population. This is also referred to as "external validity" of a study.
- *Allocation bias* occurs when the allocation of participants to the different treatment (or control) groups is systematically different. This is why comparative data at baseline are important. They are usually presented at the start of the Results section of a paper. Conformation that the groups were sufficiently similar prior to the intervention of interest will enable the reader to be more confident that any differences found after treatment can be attributed to the intervention and not to systematic differences at baseline.
- *Maturation bias* refers to changes that may have happened naturally over time rather than as a result of the intervention. This can take the form of "spontaneous" recovery in a condition that is time-limited. Maturation bias may also be seen in progressive neurological conditions where deterioration in a condition may counteract potential improvement from an intervention.
- *Attrition bias* refers to systematic and unequal numbers of participants in the different groups who withdraw or who are lost to a study. There may be many important reasons why people cease to continue in a treatment study; failure to take this into account when analysing the data may lead to spurious and misleading results.
- *Outcome measurement bias* occurs if the way that data are measured differs systematically between the groups. This is the main reason why "objective" measurement tools are preferred to "subjective" tools, as it is assumed that the latter group is more susceptible to investigator bias. The reality is rather more complicated in voice disorders, as we will discuss in Chapter 8: Techniques for measuring voice changes over time. Similarly, this is the main reason why those undertaking and assessing the outcome measurement should have no knowledge (be "blind" to) of the status of the study participants (e.g., which treatment they received or whether the measurement being performed is pre-or post-treatment).
- The *placebo effect* occurs when an improvement is noted in the participants' condition, but this improvement results from an expectation or belief that the intervention they were receiving would cause an improvement. It is perhaps difficult to apply this concept to behavioural treatments in voice disorders. It

is most commonly seen in drug trials where the control group participants report an improvement from taking a "dummy" drug because of the belief that the drug would benefit them.
- The *Hawthorne effect* occurs when participants experience improvement, or more strictly, changes (in either direction) because of the attention they are receiving as part of the research process. Obviously, for ethical reasons, research studies have to acquire consent from participants and, hence, the Hawthorne effect is a constant concern.

## Confounding factors

Confounding factors are those uncontrolled factors that may confuse the interpretation of the outcome of interest. A robust study design will identify the most likely confounding factors and eliminate them (for example, by setting participant inclusion and exclusion criteria). A major purpose of a randomised controlled trial is to spread the confounding factors randomly between the two groups and thus, eliminate their influence on the study outcomes. If these confounding variables are not randomly (and hence "evenly") distributed or controlled for, then there is a risk that one group will be "stacked" more heavily with these factors than the other. In these cases, differences between the groups cannot confidently be attributed to the intervention.

Randomisation of participants between the two (or more) treatment groups has a further significant advantage which explains its superiority as a study design. Randomisation also distributes *unknown* confounding factors – factors that the researchers were not even aware of but which could, nevertheless, influence the results. Therefore, in an intervention study, variables such as patient motivation, personal circumstances, general health, cognitive ability, life experiences and health beliefs (to name just a few) could be potential unknown confounding factors which may have an impact on treatment outcomes. Again, randomisation is the best method to "even out" these unknowns and uncontrolled factors across the treatment groups.

## External validity of a study

External validity of a study refers to the generalisability of the results to the clinical population. That is, how confidently can the clinician directly apply the results from any given study to other people with the same clinical problem? This is clearly related to the concept of selection bias addressed in the section above.

External validity is a "value" judgement, in that the reader has to determine the extent to which he believes the study population to be sufficiently representative of the general clinical population of interest.

This concept of external validity creates a problem for all clinical research. There is a constant tension between designing a study that is both scientifically robust and clinically relevant. Scientific rigour demands that the major variables are controlled in order to minimise their influence on the study results and increase our confidence that the differences are due to the intervention of interest. However, over-stringent application may result in the examination of a study population or the delivery of a treatment protocol that bears little or no resemblance to the circumstances of routine clinical practice.

## Efficacy vs effectiveness

It is important to consider the difference between treatment efficacy and treatment effectiveness in the context of this section. They are not synonymous terms. *Efficacy* refers to interventions that are tested in ideal circumstances, such as where treatment protocols are very strictly adhered to and participant selection is very specific. Efficacy has been accurately defined as "the probability of benefit to individuals in a defined population from a medical technology [i.e., a therapy intervention] applied to a given medical condition under ideal conditions of use" (Office of Technology Assessment, 1978). Robey (2004) states that in efficacy testing, "the researcher's task is to assure that only the effect of the independent variable (i.e., the treatment protocol) on the dependent variable (i.e., the clinical outcome) plausibly accounts for observed change in the outcome measured".

In contrast, *effectiveness* refers to interventions that are tested in more realistic, clinically representative situations. This has been defined as "the probability of benefit to individuals from a defined population from a medical technology applied for a given medical problem under average conditions of use" (Office of Technology Assessment, 1978). That is "the effectiveness of a treatment protocol is the expectation of benefit when it is provided in a typical fashion by typical practitioners to typical patients in typical clinical settings" (Robey, 2004) These later studies are often referred to as 'pragmatic' studies, which accommodate more typical practice and less strict procedural rigour.

Therefore, a treatment for a condition is ultimately judged by its effectiveness. However, effectiveness cannot be tested unless efficacy has been established. This forms the basis of the five-phase model described in Table 2.

### Clinical vs statistical significance

The concept of the difference between clinical and statistical significance is also important to discuss here. The determination of clinical significance is another value judgement to be made by the reader. Clinical significance is defined as "the minimum difference that would be important to a patient" (Hoffman *et al.*, 2013). For these reasons the term "clinical significance" is often used interchangeably with "clinical importance". Statistical significance is a very different concept and is described below.

## Some basic statistics

A reasonable understanding of some very basic concepts in statistics is essential when evaluating the evidence of clinical effectiveness. There are numerous high quality books on basic statistics which describe and illustrate the key concepts with clarity and relevance. One that I have found very useful is *The Handbook for Research Methods in Nursing and Health Sciences* (2nd edition) by V Minichiello (2003). Also, I highly recommend Tim Pring's book *Research Methods in Communication Disorders* (2005). The section below is a very brief overview of some of the basic concepts.

### Why bother with statistical tests at all?

In our examination of the treatment effectiveness of voice disorders we will come across many studies that present group data. It is virtually impossible to imagine that all participants in any one group in any given study will respond in exactly the same way; individual differences between subjects will inevitably occur. Treatment will not confer the same benefit to all participants in the treated group equally and some participants in the untreated (or differently treated) group will improve for reasons of their own. As mentioned above, statistical tests calculate the probability of a chance result.

### Parametric and non-parametric statistics

Researchers usually want to use parametric statistics as these are more likely to produce a statistically significant result. This is because parametric tests make some assumptions about the nature of the data. Without going into detail here (see book recommendations above), these assumptions are about the data being "normally" (symmetrically) distributed, equally variable and measured on an equal-interval scale. Non-parametric tests do not make these assumptions and are thus much more widely applicable. However, these tests are less "powerful" for producing a statistically significant result. Applied research in the behavioural sciences (e.g., voice therapy) often deals with data that are not suitable for parametric tests.

## Statistical significance

Statistical significance is a means of expressing the probability of a chance result. This is written in shorthand as the $p$ value (where the $p$ is short for "probability"). Statisticians calculate the $p$ value to establish how likely it is that the difference is due to chance alone. All $p$ values range between 1.0 (absolutely sure that the difference is due to chance alone) and 0.0 (absolutely sure that the difference is not due to chance alone). In reality these extreme values never exist and one can never be *absolutely* sure of these matters. The convention is that if $p$ is less than 0.05 ($p = <0.05$) then we can assume that chance was so unlikely that we can discount it as the cause of the difference. When the analysis of a study's results have a $p$ value <0.05, that result is considered statistically significant. By convention, when a study produces a result where the $p$ value is <0.01 (1 in a 100) then the result is considered "highly statistically significant".

## Means and standard deviation

The *mean* score (or the "average" score) is a measure of central tendency within a group of scores. It is the commonest way of describing the "typical" score in a sample. While the mean is the best measure of central tendency, it is not the only one: the "mode" is the most frequently occurring score and the "median" is the middle score. When the mean, mode and median scores are very similar we can be sure that the data are symmetrically (or "normally") distributed. Symmetrically distributed datasets are more appropriately analysed by parametric statistics (as we saw in the section above). Very "skewed" data, where the mean differs considerably from the median, is an indicator of non-symmetrical distribution and are thus more suited to non-parametric statistical analysis. The *standard deviation* is the best way of describing how the data are distributed around the mean. Standard deviation is more than just a way of describing the 'range of scores', noting just the lowest (smallest) and highest (largest) scores. Researchers rarely report individual scores (unless in a case study or case series) but will provide group means and standard deviations to show the dispersal or "spread" of the scores. These means and standard deviation scores are central to the calculation of statistical significance.

## Correlation

Correlation statistics are used to measure the relationship between variables. These data are often represented in the literature with scatterplots. Two sets of data are very unlikely to be perfectly correlated and hence, the relationship between them is tested with a correlation co-efficient to determine whether it is statistically significant or not. These data are not particularly common in treatment efficacy studies but may be used, for example, to investigate the relationship (correlation) between two different outcome measures (how well they agree with one another).

## Power calculations

A potential problem arises when a study produces results that are not statistically significant. This might mean either that there is truly no difference or that the sample was too small to detect one. This dilemma is commonly posed when the study results are "approaching statistical significance". Obviously, statistical significance can be made more likely by increasing the size of the sample (in effect, reducing the variance of the sample). A study is said to have enough "power" if it is based on sufficiently large numbers to detect sufficient meaningful difference. As Hoffman *et al.* (2010) state: "In other words, the power of a study is the degree to which we are certain that, if we conclude [from the results] that a difference does *not* exist, that it in fact does *not* exist" (page 35). The accepted level of power is conventionally set as 80% (0.80). By definition therefore, an "underpowered" study is one in which there is a non-significant difference and as such, we cannot be confident that it is a "true" finding because the sample was too small.

# References

Carding P (2000) *Evaluating Voice Therapy – Measuring the Effectiveness of Treatment.* London: Whurr Publishers.

Cook D, Mulrow C, Haynes RB (1997) Systematic reviews: synthesis of best evidence for clinical decisions. *Annals of Internal Medicine* **126**: 376–80.

Hoffman T, Bennett S and Del Mar C (2010) *Evidence-based Practice across the Health Professions* 2edn. Chatswood, NSW: Churchill Livingstone, Elsevier Australia.

Minichiello V (2003) *The Handbook for Research Methods in Nursing and Health Sciences* 2edn. Melbourne, Victoria: Pearson Australia.

Office of Technology Assessment (1978) Assessing the efficacy and safety of medical technologies. Washington, DC: US Government Printing Office.

Pring T (2005) *Research Methods in Communication Disorders.* London: Whurr.

Robey RR (2004) A five-phase model for clinical outcome research. *Journal of Communication Disorders* **37**: 401–411.

Rosenfeld RM (1995) Reading between the lines in medical journals. New Orleans LA; AAO-HNS Instruction Program **112**(5): 35.

# 3

# The effectiveness of voice therapy for functional voice disorders

## Marianne Bos-Clark and Paul Carding

### Defining functional dysphonia

Functional dysphonia is defined as a voice disturbance without structural or neurological laryngeal pathology (Roy, 2003; Boone *et al.*, 2010). Patients present with an essentially normal larynx on ENT examination and the dysphonia is primarily the result of inappropriate laryngeal muscle tension. Other terms such as "hyperfunctional", "non-organic" or "muscle tension dysphonia" (Altman *et al.*, 2005; Baker *et al.*, 2007) are considered synonymous.

The aetiology of functional dysphonia is multi-factorial and includes technical misuse, vocal strain and overuse and stress (Roy, 2008; Baker, 2008; Solomon, 2008; Oates and Winkworth 2008; Baker *et al.*, 2014). Patients can experience anxiety and depression as a result of their functional voice disorder (Caldeira *et al.*, 2015) and where psychogical stress is a primary causing and maintaining factor, patients are more accurately diagnosed with psychogenic dysphonia and treated accordingly (Butcher *et al.*, 2007; Baker *et al.* 2014).

Functional dysphonia can lead to laryngeal pathology, for example, when hyperfunctional laryngeal behaviour persists over time it can result in vocal fold nodules or vocal fold oedema. Treatment efficacy/effectiveness for vocal nodules is considered separately in Chapter 4. Many organic voice disorders also co-exist with functional dysphonia as the laryngeal musculature compensates for the primary vocal disturbance. Hyperfunction may occur, for example, as compensatory or secondary supra-glottic muscle tension with a vocal lesion or unilateral vocal fold palsy as discussed in Chapter 5 and Chapter 6, respectively. This may explain why some voice intervention studies include participants with a variety of organic and non-organic diagnoses.

This chapter will focus on primary functional dysphonia without observable organic change or significant psychological factors. This category of voice patients represents the largest proportion of patients referred to speech pathology following examination and diagnosis in the Ear, Nose and Throat (ENT) department (Van Houtte *et al.,* 2009; Roy, 2003).

## The basic principles of voice therapy

Voice therapy is the universally accepted treatment of choice for people with functional dysphonia (Wilson *et al.,* 2002; Roy, 2008). The speech pathologist's management of voice disorders is guided by advice from professional organisations such as the Royal College of Speech and Language Therapists Clinical Guidelines (Taylor-Goh, 2005) and ASHA's *Clinical Practice Guideline for the Management of Hoarseness* (Schwartz *et al.,* 2009).

The aim of voice therapy is to (a) return the patient's voice to normal or best possible within their anatomic and physiologic capabilities and (b) to satisfy the patient's occupational, social and emotional vocal needs (Aronson and Bless, 2009). In functional dysphonia, where the potential for normal voice function is considerable, the aim of intervention is invariably to resolve the voice problem fully. During treatment, it is important to maximise function during the periods of voice disturbance and to reduce limitations on participation and wellbeing. Once the voice is improved, life style and vocal habit changes will promote vocal health so that the voice improvement is maintained (Mathieson, 2001).

Joint goal setting is considered crucial to the success of voice therapy (Mathieson, 2001). This way, therapeutic goals are specific and directly relevant to the person with the voice disorder and this is likely to improve compliance and motivation and to facilitate voice change that is achieved more quickly and better maintained (Shewell, 2009; Titze and Verdolini Abbott, 2012). Mathieson describes further principles for guiding voice therapy that are all directly relevant for the management of functional dysphonia. These are: following a hierarchical treatment plan, using ongoing instrumental/perceptual monitoring and aiming for maximum improvement in minimum time (Mathieson, 2001, page 372).

# Effectiveness of voice therapy for functional dysphonia

The current literature relating to the efficacy of voice therapy is summarised in Table 1 (2000–2015). This illustrates that there are a number of Phase 3 level studies (Robey, 2004). In their meta-analysis of the literature up to 2007, Ruotsalainen *et al.,* (2009) critically appraised six randomised controlled intervention studies in functional dysphonia (Beranova *et al.,* 2003; Carding *et al.,*1999; Gillivan-Murphy *et al.,* 2005; MacKenzie *et al.,* 2001; Rattenbury *et al.,* 2004; Simberg *et al.,* 2006). They concluded that there was good evidence to support the effectiveness of direct and indirect voice therapy approaches for patients with functional dysphonia. It is also clear from Table 1 that there are a number of Phase 1 and Phase 2 studies pertaining to more "emerging" treatment techniques. These studies will be described in detail later in this chapter.

The Phase 3 studies listed below provide good evidence of treatment efficacy, using large sample sizes and (commonly) randomised controlled designs. Following the systematic review by Ruotsalainen and colleagues' (2009), several authors (Benninger, 2010; Bos-Clark and Carding, 2011) highlighted the need for additional studies that:

(a) are of high quality design
(b) use outcome measures with proven validity, reliability and sensitivity to change
(c) compare the relative benefit of different therapy approaches
(d) describe the content of voice therapy.

Three RCT studies have been published since these recommendations (Nguyen and Kenny, 2009; Rodriguez-Parra *et al.,* 2011; Wenke *et al.,* 2014). These studies attempt to meet some of the recommendations and to strengthen the evidence base further. It is also clear that there are no Phase 4 or Phase 5 (Robey, 2004) studies relating to intervention for functional voice disorders.

Table 1. Studies of Voice Treatment for Functional Dysphonia (Publications 2000–2015)

| Study | n | Type of Treatment | Outcome measures | Findings |
|---|---|---|---|---|
| **PHASE 1 studies (Robey 2004)** | | | | |
| Rubin et al., 2007 | 26 | "Physical therapy" + voice therapy | Postural ratings by two raters | 1. Subjective ratings of improvement by treating physiotherapist<br>2. No statistical analysis |
| Chen et al., 2007 | 24 mixed pathology (including FD) | Resonant voice therapy (1 x 8 weeks) | 1. Perceptual voice rating (self devised)<br>2. Laryngostroboscopy<br>3. F0 measures<br>4. VHI<br>5. Phonation threshold pressure | 1. Significant differences pre vs post in a large majority of measures |
| Van Lierde et al., 2007 | 27 | Therapy detail not given<br>Long term (6 years) follow up | 1. Perceptual voice rating (self devised)<br>2. Acoustic analysis<br>3. VHI<br>4. Dysphoniaseverity index | 1. Significant difference pre vs post :Roughness ratings ( = 0.02)<br>2. No other $p$ values given |
| Voerman et al., 2008 | 116 (including psychogenic aphonia) | Mental imagery and "laryngeal shaking" | Judgement 'cured' or 'not cured' | 1. No statistical analysis reported |
| Mathieson et al., 2009 | 10 | Laryngeal manual therapy (1 session only) | 1. Multi-dimensional voice profile<br>2. Formant frequency analysis (RAP)<br>3. Vocal tract discomfort scale<br>4. Palpatory evaluation change | 1. Significant changes pre vs post in most measures ($p = <0.05$) |
| Fischer et al., 2009 | 77 (40 controls vs 37 treat) | Intensified voice therapy | 1. German voice handicap questionnaire | 1. No significant difference between the groups |

| Study | n | Type of Treatment | Outcome measures | Findings |
|---|---|---|---|---|
| Morsomme, 2010 | 29 | Long term outcomes | 1. VAS<br>2. Perceptual voice rating-GRB<br>3. VHI10 | 1. Significant differences pre vs post for VHI-10 and Grade (g) ($p = <0.05$) |
| Kleemola et al., 2011 | 95 (mixed pathology) | Mixed intervention long term (12 months) follow-up | 1. VAPP | 1. Significant difference pre vs post ($p = <0.001$) |
| Law et al 2012 | 12 | Group voice therapy | 1. VAPP | 1. Significant differences pre vs post ($p = <0.05$) |
| McCullough et al., 2012 | 6 | Flow phonation - detailed treatment protocol | 1 Airflow measures<br>2. NHR<br>3. Perceptual voice rating - CAPE-V<br>4. VHI | 1. Significant differences for all measures (pre vs post) $p = 0.005$ |
| Watts et al., 2014 | 8 | Stretch and flow voice therapy | 1. s/z Ratio<br>2. MPT<br>3. Cepstral peak prominence<br>4. VHI | Significant change in all measures ($p = <0.05$) |
| Ogawa et al., 2014 | 41 (20 controls vs 21 FD) | "Humming" therapy | 1. Rating of roughness (only)<br>2. EGG: Closed quotient | 1. Significant difference between groups on both measures $p = <0.05$<br>2. Results are immediately after the task (only) |
| Tomlinson and Archer, 2015 | 9 | Manual therapy Detailed description of intervention | 1. Self rating scale<br>2. Patient functional scale<br>3. VHI<br>4. Standard measures of cervical and jaw range of motion | 1. Some evidence of improvement<br>2. No $p$ values reported |

# EVALUATING THE EFFECTIVENESS OF VOICE THERAPY

| Study | n | Type of Treatment | Outcome measures | Findings |
|---|---|---|---|---|
| Guzman et al., 2015 | 80 (40 control vs. 40 FD) | Semi-occluded voice exercises | EGG: Closed quotient | 1. Some specific exercises found a significant difference in CQ $p =$ <0.05<br>2. Results are immediately after the task, not generalised after time in therapy |
| Halawa et al., 2013 | 65 | Unknown | 1. Laryngoscopy<br>2. Clinician judgement of clinical improvement | 1. No correlation between laryngoscopic parameters and clinical judgement<br>2. No $p$ values reported |
| **PHASE 2 studies (Robey 2004)** | | | | |
| Ilomaki 2008 | 60 mixed pathology (including FD) | Vocal hygiene vs voice training | 1. Perceptual voice ratings (self devised)<br>2. VHI<br>3. F0measures<br>4. Jitter<br>5. Shimmer | 1. Significant differences between the two groups on most measures ($p =$ <0.05) |
| Niebudek-Bogusz et al., 2008 | 133 (53 control vs 80 treat) mixed pathology (70% FD) | Direct and indirect voice therapy Detailed description of therapy protocol | 1. MPT<br>2. Voice range<br>3. Self evaluation | 1. Significant differences between the groups on all measures ($p =$ <0.05) |
| Van Lierde et al., 2010 | 10 (5 vs 5) | Manual therapy vs vocalization and abdominal breathing therapy | 1. Dysphonia severity index | 1. Significant difference between treatment groups ($p =$ <0.001) |
| Stepp et al., 2011 | 16 (FD and vocal nodules) | No details of therapy | 1. Relative fundamental frequency | 1. Significant differences pre vs post $p =$ <0.001 |

| Study | n | Type of Treatment | Outcome measures | Findings |
|---|---|---|---|---|
| Marszalek et al., 2012 | 40 | Osteopathic myofacial techniques - Intensive treatment (1 week) | 1. Osteopath rating scale<br>2. Laryngoscopy<br>3. MPT<br>4. VHI | 1. Significant differences pre vs post $p <0.05$ on some measures |
| Mathur et al., 2015 | 15 (10 treatment, 5 no treatment) mixed diagnoses | Unknown | 1. MPT<br>2. s/z ratio<br>3. Perceptual voice ratings- CAPE-V (3 raters) | 1. Significant differences between the groups ($p = <0.05$)<br>2. No data on intra-rater reliability |
| **PHASE 3 studies (Robey, 2004)** | | | | |
| MacKenzie et al., 2001 | 133 (63 control vs 70 treatment) | A range of direct and indirect voice therapy techniques | 1. Perceptual voice rating - Buffalo Voice Profile<br>2. Jitter, shimmer<br>3. VPQ<br>4. HADS<br>5. SF36 | 1. Significant difference between the groups for perceptual rating of voice quality ($p = 0.001$) |
| Beranova and Betka, 2003 | 18 (2 treatments 9:9) | Vocal hygiene vs pharmacotherapy | 1. Phonetogram<br>2. VRQ_of L | 1. Significant differences between the groups on both measures ($p = <0.05$) |
| Rattenbury et al., 2004 | 50 (26 control vs 24 treatment) | Endoscopy Controlled therapy | 1. Perceptual voice rating-1. GRBAS<br>2. EGG<br>3. VPQ<br>4. Therapy time | 1. Significant difference between the groups of all measures ($p = <0.001$) |
| Gillivan-Murphy et al., 2005 | 20 (11 control vs 9 treatment) | Vocal function exercises | 1. VRQoL<br>2. VoiSS<br>3. Voice care knowledge score | 1. Significant difference between the groups of VoiSS and knowledge score ($p = <0.05$) |

| Study | n | Type of Treatment | Outcome measures | Findings |
|---|---|---|---|---|
| Simberg et al., 2006 | 40 (20 control vs. 20 group treatment) | Group therapy | 1. Perceptual voice rating- GRBAS<br>2. VRQoL<br>3. Laryngoscopy | 1. Significant difference between the groups for perceptual rating and VRQoL ($p = <0.05$) |
| Nguyen and Kenny, 2009 | 40 (18 control vs 22 treatment) | Vocal function exercises | 1. Jitter<br>2. Shimmer<br>3. HNR<br>4. Perceptual voice rating (anchor matching)<br>5. Self rating | 1. Significant differences between the groups on most measures ($p = <0.005$) |
| Rodriguez-Parra et al., 2011 | 42 (mixed pathology) | Voice therapy and vocal hygiene | 1. MPT<br>2. Mean Exhalation Time<br>3. Jitter<br>4. Self designed scales (well-being, self-voice, hygiene anxiety) | 1. Significant difference pre vs post on some measures ($p = <0.05$) |
| Wenke et al., 2014 | 16 | Intensive vs standard weekly therapy | 1. VHI<br>2. Australian therapy outcome measures | Significant difference in VHI ($p = 0.003$)<br>No significant difference in AusTOMS |

Note: $F_0$ = fundamental frequency; PTP = phonation threshold pressure; VI = vocal intensity; MPT = maximum phonation time; RAP = relative average perturbation; PPQ = pitch perturbation quotient; SPL = speech pressure level; EGG = electroglottography; VPQ = Vocal Performance Questionnaire; VHI = Voice Handicap Index; SNL = spectral noise level; HNR = Harmonics to Noise Ratio; VRQoL = Voice Related Quality of Life Questionnaire; EGG = Electroglottography (Laryngography); HADS = Hospital Anxiety and Depression Scale; VAPP = Voice Activity Participation Profile.

# Efficacy from non-RCT intervention studies (emerging treatments)

Table 1 (above) illustrates that the evidence base for voice therapy interventions for functional dysphonia has continued to grow with respect to innovative and different treatment modalities. This is particularly true in the examination of the efficacy of manual laryngeal therapies and flow phonation therapy, or semi-occluded vocal tract therapy (SOVT).

## Manual therapies (laryngeal palpation therapies)

A range of palpation methods used in the assessment and treatment of muscle tension dysphonia is described in the literature (Rubin et al., 2007; Lieberman, 1998). However, all are yet to demonstrate clear validity and reliability (Roy, 2008; Khoddami et al., 2015). Nevertheless, various studies suggest that manual therapy is likely to be beneficial in the treatment of functional dysphonia (Mathieson, 2011).

Rubin et al., (2007) described an initial case series of 26 dysphonic professional voice users with musculoskeletal problems, who appeared to benefit from laryngeal "physical therapy" in combination with other interventions. A subsequent study by Mathieson et al., (2009) found further positive evidence for the use of laryngeal manual therapy in the treatment of muscle tension dysphonia. After only one session, Mathieson et al., (2009) reported improved acoustic measures and reduced severity and frequency of vocal tract discomfort in 10 patients with muscle tension dysphonia. Van Lierde et al., (2010) reported a study comparing the effects of manual circumlaryngeal therapy and vocalization with abdominal breath support. Statistically significant improvement in overall voice quality was found following manual therapy only, suggesting this is an effective technique for patients with laryngeal muscle tension (Van Lierde et al., 2010). Similarly, Tomlinson and Archer (2015) reported a recent case series which found apparent benefits from a mixed intervention (including manual therapy) in patients with muscle tension dysphonia and infer appropriate implications about clinical application and the need for more methodologically robust controlled studies.

Methodologically weaker studies by Voerman et al., (2008) and Marszalek et al., (2012) combine manual therapies with other interventions such as voice exercises and stress management counselling. Whilst results suggested that these combined therapies are beneficial in functional dysphonia, many variables remained uncontrolled and it is not possible to determine the relative value of each.

These recent pilot studies and small comparative case series have contributed significantly to the development of an early evidence base for manual therapy intervention in functional dysphonia. They provide valuable preliminary data for power calculations, use of outcome measures and procedure for the development of further, larger, controlled studies (Robey, 2004). In a comprehensive review of the evidence base for laryngeal manual therapies in the treatment of muscle tension dysphonia, Mathieson (2011) called for further intervention research using high quality designs to determine the efficacy of manual therapies in the treatment of functional dysphonia. To date, no such trial has been published.

## Flow phonation therapy (semi-occluded vocal tract therapy: SOVT).

A range of established and well described therapy programmes use the principles of a semi-occluded vocal tract (Titze, 2006; Story *et al.*, 2000). These programmes include *Lessac-Madsen Resonant Voice Therapy* (Verdolini, 2008), Stemple's *Vocal Function Excercises* (Stemple *et al.*, 2010) and *The Accent Method* (Thyme-Frokjaer and Frokjaer-Jensen, 2001). Flow phonation or semi-occluded vocal tract therapy is based on partial closure of the filter to change resistance to the airflow and establishing a level of back pressure on the vocal folds, generally with the aim to produce phonation with less effort (Simberg and Laine, 2007; Titze, 2006; Story *et al.*, 2000). A number of different semi-occluded or flow exercises are described in the literature (Behrman and Haskell, 2008; Andrade *et al.*, 2014), many of which have long been a part of traditional voice therapy or singing training. Recent research has sought to describe the physiological effects within the larynx (Andrade *et al.*, 2015; Granqvist *et al.*, 2014; Gaskill and Quinney, 2011; Enflo *et al.*, 2012; Dargin and Searl, 2014) in an effort to predict the effect on phonation of specific exercises and different conditions (e.g., diameter and length of straw, in/out of water, depth of water). Most of these studies use very small groups of participants with normal voices (often singers) and measure outcome with a wide range of instruments. In their article on the resonance tube method in voice therapy, Simberg and Laine (2007) provide a clear overview of the clinical application of this work and call for research studies into the effectiveness of this mode of voice therapy. Recent well-designed research has examined the specific effects of semi-occluded interventions in hyperfunctional dysphonia in an experimental setting (Paes *et al.*, 2013; Guzman *et al.*, 2013; Guzman *et al.*, 2015).

Few studies have examined the effects of flow phonation therapy in a clinical population. In a well-designed pilot study, McCullough *et al.* (2012) reported the effects of three specific flow phonation exercises on a small number of participants with hyperfunctional dysphonia ($n = 6$, no control). Two of the four outcome measures showed a statistically significant difference following treatment. In a prospective case series, Watts *et al.* (2014) also reported preliminary efficacy evidence of flow phonation therapy, this time in eight patients with primary muscle tension dysphonia and phonotraumatic lesions due to hyperfunctional behaviours. Both studies concluded that further research with more rigorous methodology and larger numbers is warranted.

The SOVT approaches appear to have a significant body of laboratory-based scientific evidence to claim "proof of concept" and hence justify the call for improved scientific evaluation of intervention effectiveness. It is hoped that these basic science foundations will accelerate the progression of a sound clinical evidence base from the current Phase1 (Robey, 2004) level in the near future.

## Other intervention programmes

A small number of recent studies has investigated the benefit of other specific interventions in functional dysphonia. These intervention programmes include vocal function exercises, humming exercises and resonance therapy.

Chen *et al.*, (2007) reported on 24 female teachers participating in an eight-week resonant voice therapy programme. While the intervention appears standardised and common outcome measures are used, the lack of a control group and the heterogeneous nature of underlying pathology limit the conclusions that can be drawn from this study. Ngyen *et al.*, (2009) detailed a randomised controlled trial with a small group of female teachers with functional dysphonia. Treatment variables appear well controlled and voice outcomes show statistically significant changes following a specific and detailed Vocal Function Exercises programme. Ogawa *et al.*, (2014) found a statistically significant improvement in glottal contact measures following "humming" therapy in a group of patients with muscle tension dysphonia. The benefits of this technique appear promising and represent initial proof of concept which requires more detailed investigation.

Over the past decade, a number of other voice therapy intervention studies have included participants with functional dysphonia along with other types of voice disorders. For example Rodriguez-Parra *et al.* (2011) evaluated intervention to a group of dysphonic speakers with wide-ranging pathologies including hypotonic dysphonia, angiomatous polyps, Reinke's oedema and nodules. More commonly, studies have included patients with and without observable organic changes in the larynx, often because the focus of the research is occupational groups rather than diagnostic categories such as teachers (Martins *et al.*, 2014; Ziegler *et al.*, 2010; Chen *et al.*, 2007). Niebudek-Bogusz *et al.* (2008) described how 133 teachers with a range of diagnosed pathologies responded to voice training consisting of a mixture of direct and indirect approaches. Ilomaki *et al* (2008) and Mathur *et al.* (2015) similarly reported the results of an intervention to a heterogeneous group of teachers. These studies support the effectiveness of a combination of direct and indirect intervention found in other (earlier) studies which have had the benefit of diagnostic homogeneity and methodological rigour.

## Other significant developments in the evidence base

There have been some other significant developments in the quality of the evidence base for the treatment of functional dysphonia since the systematic review by Ruotsalainen *et al.*(2009). These developments include: (1) assessment and outcome measurement, (2) therapy content, (3) therapy delivery (intensity/doseage) and (4) long term outcomes. These are discussed in detail below.

### Assessment and outcome measurement

Multi-dimensional evaluation of voice is widely supported by the literature (Speyer *et al.*, 2004; Welham, 2009; Carding *et al.*, 2009). In a systematic review of evidence-based clinical voice assessment, Roy *et al.*, (2012) called for further high quality research into what should form part of standard clinical voice assessment. Since the aetiology of functional dysphonia is multi-factorial, assessment needs to be systematic, use instrumental and perceptual measures and consider the impact of certain variables on individual patients in the context of their lives (Roy *et al.*, 2012). Carding *et al.*, (2009) reviewed three main areas of outcome measurement: acoustic assessment; patient self-report; and perceptual voice rating. Their findings are discussed with others in the relevant sections below.

## Laryngeal examination

Sama *et al.*, (2001) found that laryngoscopic characteristics associated with functional dysphonia are also common in the normal population and therefore cannot always distinguish between them. However, detailed examination of phonatory physiology, with and without stroboscopy, provides useful observations of inefficient laryngeal function such as supra-glottic constriction, bowing, or large glottic chink. With both technological advances and expansion of the role of the voice specialist SLT in recent years, detailed laryngeal examinations are more commonplace in voice therapy clinical practice (Jones, 2016). These observations can serve as an outcome measure as well as a means of helping to design therapy (Carding, 2013; Rattenbury and Carding, 2004; Jones, 2016).

Halawa *et al.*, (2013) evaluated the effectiveness of laryngostroboscopy in functional dysphonia in 65 patients. Of the four laryngoscopic parameters, glottal closure, fold vibration, mucosal wave and phase symmetry, only improvement in glottal closure post-therapy was statistically significant. The other parameters did not correlate with perceptual improvement following therapy and the authors conclude that in functional dysphonia, laryngostroboscopy is more useful in diagnosis than in treatment outcome measurement.

Laryngoscopic assessment is a subjective observer judgement. In a systematic review of rater methodology for stroboscopy, Bonilha *et al.*, (2014) found only 2 of 11 studies report good inter- and intra-rater reliability. Overall, the rating of anatomical rather than functional features was more reliable (Bonilha *et al.*, 2014; Beaver, 2003). Voigt *et al.*, (2010) reported the development of a computer-aided method to increase the reliability of the diagnosis of functional voice disorder. Results suggested that objective analysis of dysfunctional vocal fold vibration can be achieved with high accuracy. No further studies have followed.

## Acoustic analysis

Commercial acoustic analysis packages and free downloadable software such as PRAAT (Madill and McCabe, 2011), provide measurements of regularity of vocal fold closure, pitch (Jitter) and loudness (Shimmer) that may be used as outcome measures for treatment. However, Carding *et al.*, (2009) concluded that there is insufficient evidence of reliability or sensitivity to change in these techniques to measure change over time. Brockmann-Hauser and Drinnan (2011) similarly reviewed recent evidence regarding acoustic voice analysis; they concluded that its validity in clinical applications remains unproven and that reliability is limited. They suggested that acoustic analysis may have value in outcome measurement as long as measurement protocols are followed and variables such as gender, vowel and vocal intensity are controlled (Brockmann-Bauser and Drinnan, 2011). The adherence to such stringent protocols has not, on the whole, been observed in recent intervention studies.

Preliminary data on OperaVOX, a mobile device voice analysis programme, suggested that reliability is equivalent to that of a commonly used acoustic analysis package (Mat Baki *et al.*, 2015).

## Patient-reported symptoms

Symptom-based questionnaires that link to a patient's quality of life have been found to provide a valid and reliable outcome measurement in evaluation of the effectiveness of therapy in functional dysphonia. Carding *et al.*, (2009) reviewed the reliability, validity and sensitivity of several common patient report tools and recommended the use of the Vocal Performance Questionnaire (Carding and Horsley 1992) or the VHI-10 (Rosen *et al.*, 2004). Branski *et al.*, (2010) appraised nine different questionnaires used with dysphonic speakers. They concluded that the Vocal Symptom Index (Deary *et al.*, 2003) was the most psychometrically robust and content valid. They reported that the content validity of VoiSS enabled more accurate recording of the variables that appear to be the most important to people with voice disorders. Laukkannen *et al.*, (2009) highlighted the limitations of the use of self-evaluation of voice as a treatment outcome measure due to the potential placebo effect and the patients' inclination to "please" the clinician/researcher.

## Perceptual evaluation of voice quality

Oates (2009) considered the advantages and drawbacks of auditory-perceptual evaluation and makes relevant suggestions for its use in clinical evaluation. The GRBAS scale (Hirano, 1981) is widely used and is suggested as a minimum standard for clinical practice (Carding *et al.*, 2009). Inter-rater reliability of the GRBAS scale on sustained vowels and counting tasks in high, habitual and low registers are found to have the highest reliability (Lu and Matteson, 2014). The CAPE-V scale, developed from the GRBAS scale, is a more sensitive measure with equally good reliability (Karnell *et al.*, 2007). Nemr *et al.*, (2012) showed that both GRBAS and CAPE-V scales provide reliable data and are thus recommended as valuable measures of change post-voice therapy. It is important to consider that even when studies use common outcome measures, they may not have been used in a similar way. For example, Halawa *et al.*, (2013) reported an improvement following therapy as a binary yes–no judgement by the ENT and SLT, based on perceptual assessment with GRBAS in which they refer to a seven-point scale instead of the usual four-point voice quality rating scale.

## Palpation rating scales

Several clinician rating scales can be used to denote perceived levels of muscular tension, larynx height and other observations (Mathieson *et al.*, 2009; Angsuwarangsee and Morrison, 2012), but little is known about their validity and inter- and intra-rater reliability at this stage (Khoddami *et al.*, 2015).

Lowell *et al.* (2012) used Mathieson's manual therapy rating scale in their detailed radiographic study of hyoid position, laryngeal position and hyolaryngeal space in 10 patients with muscle tension dysphonia compared with normal speakers. They found no correlation between larynx position subscore and radiographic measurement and low to moderate correlation between the overall rating and radiographic hyoid and laryngeal position.

## Other instrumental outcome measures

Van Houtte *et al.*, (2013) examined surface EMG in assessment of muscle tension and concluded that this is not a useful tool; they found no significant difference in sEMG values between people with and without muscle tension dysphonia. Stepp *et al.*, (2011) suggested that Relative Fundamental Frequency (RFF) may be a useful acoustic outcome measure and report RFF measures in patients with vocal hyperfunction after therapy that are similar to those seen in individuals with a healthy voice ($n = 16$). However, a subsequent study found a weak negative correlation with perceptual evaluation of vocal effort (Stepp *et al.*, 2012). Ogawa's study of the effectiveness of humming therapy found that electroglottography (EGG) increased regularity of vocal fold vibration and improved glottal contact.

It is clear that a wide range of outcome measures is reported within the literature, as illustrated by Table 1. The fact that intervention studies use such a range of outcome measures with variable levels of proven validity, reliability and sensitivity to change complicates comparative judgement of the research. This issue is discussed further in Chapter 8.

## Therapy content and delivery

Voice therapy for functional dysphonia consists of a potentially wide variety of activities and can be delivered in different formats. Clinical practice varies depending on patient, clinician and service provider factors. In the delivery of voice therapy, "no single technique will be equally effective with all individuals" (Colton *et al.*, 2011, page 326) and it is therefore the constant challenge for the clinician to find the appropriate techniques to facilitate each individual's voice and to match clinical rationale with research evidence.

### Direct vs indirect therapy

It is recommended that voice therapy for functional dysphonia offers a combination of indirect and direct intervention approaches (Taylor-Goh, 2005; Enderby *et al.*, 2009; Ruoatsalainen *et al.*, 2009). Direct therapy involves specific, targeted work to control and coordinate the various aspects of the vocal system (Carding, 2000). Indirect voice therapy focuses on enabling the patient to modify the contributory and maintaining aspects of the voice disorder and includes voice education, voice care advice and stress management. To a voice clinician it may be self-evident that where the voice problem is due primarily to inappropriate muscle tension, the solution lies in clinical approaches that address this muscular imbalance. Where vocal load, lifestyle issues and psychological stress associated with dysphonia are significant factors, this direct muscular/technical work would need to be accompanied by indirect approaches that facilitate change in these domains.

Based on Carding (2000) and Gartner-Schmidt *et al.*, (2012), Table 2 lists different activities described in the literature as direct or indirect intervention. This is not an exhaustive account of all possible activities, but serves to provide examples of each.

## Table 2: Examples of Direct and Indirect Techniques or Treatment Approaches

| Indirect Voice Therapy Techniques | Direct Voice Therapy Techniques |
|---|---|
| Patient education of normal voice production and diagnosis | Facilitative techniques (yawn–sigh, pitch variation, loudness reduction) |
| Voice care advice (including hydration) | Resonant voice |
| Reassurance and psychosocial counselling | Flow phonation or semi-occluded vocal tract |
| Modification of environment Including amplification | Laryngeal manual therapy |
| General relaxation techniques | Vocal function exercises |
| General body posture work | Accent method |
| Breath work without voicing | Estill- or Voicecraft-based therapy |
| Discussion of progress and homework tasks | Generalisation activities (transfer to connected speech, projection etc.) |

The literature considers the relative benefits of direct and indirect treatment activities. In a systematic review of the effects of voice therapy, Speyer (2008) concluded that direct intervention was more effective than indirect therapy alone. In a study by Behrman *et al.*, (2008) two-thirds of patients who received direct intervention achieved a "within normal limits" score on the Voice Handicap Index, compared with only one-third in the indirect group. Rodriguez-Parra *et al.*, (2011) similarly found that voice measures were significantly better following direct intervention compared with indirect therapy. Gartner-Schmidt *et al.*, (2012) reported that speech pathologists spent three-quarters of their time using direct intervention strategies. The study also concluded that direct therapy was implemented in a similar way across different voice disorder types, while indirect therapy elements varied depending on individual and voice diagnosis, particularly in patients with functional dysphonia.

In their Cochrane review of voice therapy specific to functional dysphonia, Ruotsalainen *et al.*, (2009) concluded that a combination of direct and indirect therapy is recommended. In a study involving 45 patients with functional dysphonia, Carding *et al.*, (1999) found that 46% of patients significantly improved their voice quality with indirect therapy alone as compared with a control group and 93% of patients improved with a combination of direct and indirect intervention. In a randomised controlled trial, a combination of direct and indirect therapy was found to be effective in patients with functional dysphonia (MacKenzie *et al.*, 2001). By noting and categorising therapy activities every 5 minutes during a session, the team catalogued the content of therapy. Overall, two-thirds of therapy time was spent on indirect therapy activities and one-third of the time in direct intervention (Sellars *et al.*, 2002).

Interestingly, in a study of patients with functional dysphonia and perception of therapy, voice exercises (direct therapy) were cited by 74% of patients as the most useful aspect of voice therapy (Ziegler *et al.*, 2014).

## Therapy programme details

Recent intervention studies have provided increased detail about the content of therapy. While there is no single, systematic framework for categorising content, as suggested by Dejonckere *et al.* (2001), description of intervention in some studies does allow for some level of replication. Chen *et al.* (2007) used a specific programme of therapy, the Resonance Therapy Treatment Protocol (Verdolini Abbott, 2008). Some studies provide a very detailed description of their intervention, for example Niebudek-Bogusz *et al.*, (2008), while others fail to describe intervention to the extent that it could be replicated (Halawa *et al.*, 2013; Mathur *et al.*, 2015). From these two studies it is only possible to make broad statements of the proportion of indirect versus direct treatment approaches.

Further efficacy studies where therapy content is systematically described and analysed are needed before we can specify the most effective division of therapy time across indirect or direct intervention for patients with functional dysphonia.

## Intensity of therapy delivery

Considerable variety exists in terms of therapy intensity (Bos-Clark and Carding, 2011; De Bodt *et al.*, 2015). In the functional dysphonia intervention studies considered here, patients may attend one session (Mathieson *et al.*, 2009), or up to 73 (Van Lierde *et al.*, 2007) over a time span of a day, a week (Marzalek *et al.*, 2012; Patel *et al.*, 2011) or up to two years (Van Lierde *et al.*, 2007). With many studies reporting session averages of 45 minutes each and variability in intensity of delivery, little is known about the optimum dosage of voice therapy for this type of voice disorder.

It is suggested that intensive delivery of voice therapy is beneficial (Fischer *et al.*, 2009; Patel *et al.*, 2011). An important recent study by Wenke *et al.* (2014) evaluated the impact of intensive (4 x 1 hour a week) versus standard voice therapy (1 x 1 hour a week) in patients with functional dysphonia. After 8 hours of therapy, patients in the intensive group reported statistically significant improvements in voice symptoms and a higher level of satisfaction with their treatment. In a pragmatic randomised controlled trial, Fu *et al.*, (2015) similarly reported comparable benefits from intensive versus traditional voice therapy for patients with vocal nodules (this study is reported in more detail in the next chapter). Further research into optimal dose–response in voice therapy for functional dysphonia is needed (Roy *et al.*, 2012).

## "Teletherapy" delivery

Advances in technology have increased the levels of intensity and variety of modes in which voice therapy can be delivered. Mobile devices or computer-based support for patients in their homework tasks between sessions (King *et al.*, 2012; van Leer and Connor, 2011), computer program-based delivery of therapy tasks (Nguyen *et al.*, 2009) and "teletherapy" (delivery of therapy via computer links such as Skype) are increasingly common. Further research is needed to establish how this contributes to effectiveness of treatment and other methods of delivery.

## Group vs individual therapy

In their controlled trial of voice intervention, Simberg *et al.*, (2006) demonstrated the benefit of group intervention. A comparison of group vs traditional one-to-one voice therapy is reported by Law *et al.*, (2012). In their small case series, they found that 12 teachers with hyperfunctional dysphonia achieved statistically significant improvements on voice-related quality of life and vocal symptoms scores. Specific benefits of group interventions cited are psychosocial, clinical and health resource allocation factors. Other studies reporting group intervention also include teachers (Chen *et al.*, 2007; Ilomaki *et al.*, 2008; Pasa *et al.*, 2007), though some of these are preventative rather than specific treatment programmes.

It is clear that there are a wide number of variables associated with the content and delivery of voice therapy for functional voice disorders. The "how" of therapy in terms of the language, instructions and feedback used to facilitate vocal improvement (Titze and Verdolini, 2013; Gaskill and Quinney, 2012) warrants considerable further investigation. It is likely that specific patient and therapist factors also impact on the effectiveness of intervention. These individual therapist and patient variables are poorly understood and yet may be key to successful intervention (and key to the development of a skilled voice therapist). In recent times, more research is focused on patient factors (Smith *et al.*, 2010; Portone-Maira *et al.*, 2011) and seeking out the patients' perspective of voice therapy (Van Leer *et al.*, 2010; Da Costa *et al.*, 2012; Ziegler *et al.*, 2014). These investigative studies provide the starting point for a deeper understanding of voice therapy dynamics.

## Long term follow-up

Functional dysphonia may be recurrent and result in secondary organic complications (Baker *et al.*, 2007); therefore examination of the long-term effectiveness of voice therapy is important. Morsomme *et al.*, (2010) found that on a six-month follow-up of 29 patients with functional dysphonia, 76% reported that voice therapy benefits were maintained. Based on the patients' judgements of their voice quality and symptoms rating, the authors conclude that voice therapy plays an important role in the long-term treatment of functional dysphonia. Leppanen *et al.*, (2010) reported that improved vocal well-being was maintained at the 6- and 12-month follow-up of a group of teachers. Kleemola *et al.*, (2011) detailed maintenance of therapy benefit in 50% of patients at 12 months (as reported by the Voice Activity Participation Profile). However, in a study of 27 patients with muscle tension dysphonia six years after completion of intervention, Van Lierde *et al.* (2007) found that 51% continued to present with pathological features on laryngoscopy and that overall hoarseness was unchanged.

It is clear that this is a significant area for future research. These future studies also need to consider the inclusion of a range of outcome measures. However, there is no clear evidence base as to which outcome measures may provide the most robust data for long-term treatment effects of therapy of functional dysphonia.

## Conclusions

This review of recent research and evidence base in functional dysphonia has outlined advances in our knowledge since the 2007 Cochrane review (Ruotsalainen *et al.*, 2009). More is known about the benefits of specific interventions and about variables that impact on the efficacy of voice therapy. While a number of well-designed studies have been identified, there is a continued need for further research in speech pathology intervention for functional dysphonia. The main areas identified in the research evidence to be addressed in future research include

- reliability, validity and sensitivity of outcome measures for long-term outcome measurement
- comparative benefits of different direct treatment approaches
- treatment content, dosage and mode of delivery studies
- patient variables and perspective on intervention
- large scale effectiveness studies to determine intervention benefit in clinical practice
- cost-effectiveness studies (both in terms of fiscal and societal benefits).

# References

Altman KW, Atkinson C, Lazarus C (2005) Current and emerging concepts in muscle tension dysphonia: a 30 month review. *Journal of Voice* **19**: 261–267.

Andrade PA, Wood G, Ratcliffe P *et al*. (2014) Electroglottographic study of seven semi-occluded exercises: LaxVox, straw, lip-trill, tongue-trill, humming, hand-over-mouth and tongue-trill combined with hand-over-mouth. *Journal of Voice* **28**(5): 589–595.

Andrade PA, Wistbacka G, Larsson H *et al*. (2015) The flow and pressure relationships in different tubes commonly used for semi-occluded vocal tract exercises. *Journal of Voice* **30**(1): 36–41.

Angsuwarangsee T, Morrison M (2012) Extrinsic laryngeal muscular tension in patients with voice disorders. *Journal of Voice* **16**: 333–343.

Aronson AE, Bless DM (2009) Treatment of voice disorders. In: Aronson AE, Bless DM (Eds) *Clinical Voice Disorders* (4edn). New York, NY Thieme, pp231–270.

Benninger MS (2010) Levels of evidence on the voice literature. *Journal of Voice* **25**(6): 653–656.

Baker J, Ben-Tovim DI, Butcher A *et al*. (2007) Development of a modified diagnostic classification system for voice disorders with inter-rater reliability study. *Logopedics Phoniatrics Vocology* **32**: 99–112.

Baker J, Oates JM, Leeson E *et al*. (2014) Patterns of emotional expression and responses to health and illness in women with functional voice disorders (MTVD) and a comparison group. *Journal of Voice* **28**(6): 762–769.

Baker J (2008) The role of psychogenic and psychosocial factors in the development of functional voice disorders. *International Journal of Speech-Language Pathology* **10**: 210–230.

Beaver ME, Stasney CR, Weitzel E (2003) Diagnosis of laryngopharyngeal reflux disease with digital imaging. *Otolarygology Head and Neck Surgery* **128**: 103–108.

Behrman A, Rutledge J, Hembree A, Sheridan S (2008) Vocal hygiene education, voice production therapy and the role of patient adherence: a treatment effectiveness study in women with phonotrauma. *Journal of Speech Hearing and Language Research* **51**: 350–366.

Behrman A, Haskell J (2011) *Exercises for Voice Therapy*. San Diego, CA: Plural Publishing, Inc.

Beranova A, Betka J (2003) New opportunities in the treatment of dysphonia. *Otorinolaryngology a Foniatrie* **52**: 75–79.

Bonilha HS, Focht KL, Martin-Harris B (2014) Rater methodology for stroboscopy: a systematic review. *Journal of Voice* **29**(1): 101–108.

Boone DR, McFarlane SC, Von Berg SL et al. (2010) Functional voice disorders. In: Boone DR, McFarlane SC, Von Berg SL et al. (Eds) *The Voice and Voice Therapy* (8edn). Boston, MA: Pearson, pp113–132.

Bos-Clark M, Carding PN (2011) Effectiveness of voice therapy in functional dysphonia: where are we now? *Current Opinion in Otolaryngology and Head and Neck Surgery* **19**: 160–164.

Branski RC, Cukier-Blaj S, Pusic A et al. (2010) Measuring quality of life in dysphonic patients: a systematic review of content development in patient-reported outcome measures. *Journal of Voice* **24**: 193–198.

Brockmann-Bauser M, Drinnan MJ (2011) Routine acoustic voice analysis: time to think again? *Current Opinion in Otoloaryngology and Head and Neck Surgery* **19**: 165–170.

Butcher P, Elias A, Cavalli L (2007) *Understanding and Treating Psychogenic Voice Disorder* London: Wiley.

Caldeira Martinez C, Cassol M (2015) Measurement of voice quality, anxiety and depression symptoms after speech therapy. *Journal of Voice* **9**(4): 446–449.

Carding PN (2000) *Evaluating Voice Therapy: Measuring the Effectiveness of Treatment* London: Whurr Publishers.

Carding PN (2013) Current issues in voice assessment and intervention in the United Kingdom. In: Yiu EML(Ed) *International Perspectives on Voice Disorders* Bristol: CDAL, pp83–89.

Carding PN, Horsley IA (1992) An evaluation study of voice therapy in non-organic dysphonia. *European Journal of Disorders of Communication* **27**: 137–158.

Carding PN, Horsley IA, Docherty GJ (1999) A study of the effectiveness of voice therapy in the treatment of 45 patients with nonorganic dysphonia. *Journal of Voice* **13**(1): 72–104.

Carding PN, Wilson JA, MacKenzie K et al. (2009) Measuring voice outcomes: state of the science review. *Journal of Laryngology and Otology*. **123**: 823–829.

Chen SH, Hsiao T, Hsiao L et al. (2007) Outcome of resonant voice therapy for female teachers with voice disorders: perceptual, physiological, acoustic, aerodynamic and functional measurements. *Journal of Voice* **21**(4): 415–425.

Colton RH, Casper JK, Leonard R (2011) *Understanding Voice Problems: A Physiological Perspective for Diagnosis and Treatment* (4edn). London: Wolters Kluwer, Lippincott Williams *and* Wilkins.

Dargin TC, Searl J (2014) Semi-occluded vocal tract exercises: aerodynamic and electroglottographic measurements in singers. *Journal of Voice* 29(2): 155–164.

Da Costa V, Prada E, Roberts A, Cohen S (2012) Voice disorders in primary school teachers and barriers to care. *Journal of Voice* 26(1): 69–76.

Deary I, Wilson JA, Carding PN (2003) VoiSS: a patient-derived voice symptom scale. *Journal of Psychosomatic Research* 54: 483–489.

Dejonckere PH, Wieneke GH (2001) Basic elements in voice therapy. In: *Occupational Voice - Care and Cure* Dejonckere PH (Ed). Amsterdam: Kugler Publications, pp155–163.

De Bodt M, Patteeuw T, Versele A (2015) Temporal variables in voice therapy. *Journal of Voice* 29(5): 611–617.

Enderby P (2009) *RCSLT Resource Manual*. London: Royal College of Speech and Language Therapists.

Enflo L, Sundberg J, Romedahl C, McAllister A (2012) Effects on vocal fold collision and phonation threshold pressure of resonance tube phonation with tube end in water. *Journal of Speech Language and Hearing Research*. 56: 1530–1538.

Fischer MJ, Gutenbrunner C, Ptok M (2009) Intensified voice therapy: a new model for the rehabilitation of patients suffering from functional dysphonia. *International Journal of Rehabilitation Research*. 32: 348–355.

Fu S, Theodoros D, Ward EC (2015) Intensive versus traditional voice therapy for vocal nodules: perceptual, physiological, acoustic and aerodynamic changes. *Journal of Voice* 29(2): 260–273.

Gartner-Schmid JL, Roth DF, Zullo TG, Rosen CA (2012) Quantifying component parts of indirect and direct voice therapy related to different voice disorders. *Journal of Voice* 26(2): 1–7.

Gaskill CS, Quinney DM (2011) The effect of resonance tubes on glottal contact quotient with and without task instruction: a comparison of trained and untrained voices. *Journal of Voice* 26(3): 79–93.

Gillivan-Murphy P, Drinnan M, O'Dwyer TP et al. (2005) The effectiveness of a voice treatment approach for teachers with self-reported voice problems. *Journal of Voice*. 20(3): 423–31.

Granqvist S, Simberg S, Hertegard S et al. (2014) Resonance-tube phonation in water: high-seed imaging, electroglottographic and oral pressure observations of vocal fold vibrations: a pilot study. *Logopedics, Phoniatrics Vocology*. 2: 1–9.

Guzman M, Castro C, Testart A et al. (2013) Laryngeal and pharyngeal activity during semioccluded vocal tract postures in subjects diagnosed with hyperfunctional dysphonia. *Journal of Voice* 27(6): 709–716.

Guzman M, Calvache C, Romero L et al. (2015) Do different semi-occluded voice exercises affect vocal fold adduction differently in subjects diagnosed with hyperfunctional dysphonia? *Folia Phoniatrica et Logopaedica* (2): 68–75.

Halawa WE, Vasquez-Minoz I, Perez, SS (2013) Effectiveness of laryngostroboscopy for monitoring the evolution of functional dysphonia after rehabilitator treatment. *Indian Journal of Otolaryngology Head and Neck Surgery* 65(4): 322–326.

Hirano M (1981) *Clinical Examination of Voice*. New York, NY: Springer-Verlag.

Ilomaki I, Laukkanen AM, Leppanen K, Vilkman E (2008) Effects of voice training and voice hygiene education on acoustic and perceptual speech parameters and self-reported vocal well-being in female teachers. *Logopedics Phoniatrics Vocology* 33: 83–92.

Jones SM (2016) *Laryngeal Endoscopy and Voice Therapy: A Clinical Guide*. Oxford: Compton Publishing.

Karnell MP, Melton SD, Childres *et al.* (2007) Reliability of clinician-based (GRBAS and CAPE-V) and patient-based (V-RQOL and IPVI) documentation of voice disorders. *Journal of Voice* 21(5): 576–590.

King SN, Davis L, Lehman JH, Ruddy BH (2012) A model for treating voice disorders in school-age children in a videogaming environment. *Journal of Voice* 26(5): 656–663.

Khoddami SM, Ansari NN, Jalaie S (2015) Review on laryngeal palpation methods in muscle tension dysphonia: Validity and reliability issues. *Journal of Voice* 29(4): 459–468.

Kleemola L, Helminen M, Rorarius E *et al.* (2011) Twelve-month clinical follow-up study of voice patients' recovery using the voice activity and participation profile (VAPP). *Journal of Voice* 25(5): 245–254.

Law T, Lee KYS, Ho FNY *et al.* (2012) The effectiveness of group voice therapy: a group climate perspective. *Journal of Voice* 26(2): 41–48.

Laukkanen A, Leppanen K, Ilomaki I (2009) Self-evaluation of voice as a treatment outcome measure. *Folia Phoniatrica Logopaedica* 61: 57–65.

Leppanen K, Ilomaki I, Laukkanen, A (2010) One-year follow-up study of self-evaluated effects of Voice massage, voice training and voice hygiene lecture in female teachers. *Logopedics, Phoniatrics, Vocology* 35: 13–18.

Lieberman J (1998) Principles and techniques of manual therapy: application in the management of dysphonia. In: TM Harris, SJ Harris, JS Rubin, DM Howard (Eds) *The Voice Clinic Handbook* London: Whurr Publishers, pp91–138.

Lowell SY, Kelley RT, Colton RH *et al.* (2012) Position of the hyoid and larynx in people with muscle tension dysphonia. *Laryngoscopy* 122: 370–377.

Lu F, Matteson S (2014) Speech tasks and interrrater reliability in perceptual voice evaluation. *Journal of Voice* 28(6): 725–732.

MacKenzie K, Millar A, Wilson JA *et al.* (2001) Does voice therapy work? A randomised control trail of the efficacy of voice therapy for dysphonia. *British Medical Journal* 323; 658–661.

Madill C, McCabe P (2011) Acoustic analysis using freeware: PRAAT. In: Ma EPM and Yiu EML *Handbook of Voice Assessments* San Diego, CA: Plural Publishing, Inc, pp231–251.

Martins RHG, Pereira ERBN, Hidalgo CB, Tavares ELM (2014) Voice disorders in teachers: a review *Journal of Voice* 28(6): 716–724.

Marszalek S, Niebudek-Bogusz E, Wozniki E *et al.* (2012) Assessment of the influence of osteopathic myofascial techniques on normalization of the vocal tract functions in patients with occupational dysphonia. *International Journal of Occupational Medicine and Environmental Health* 25(3): 225–235.

Mat Baki M, Wood G, Alston M et al. (2015) Reliability of OPeraVOX against Multidimensional Voice Program. *Clinical Otolaryngology* **40**(1): 22–28.

Mathieson L (2011) The evidence for laryngeal manual therapies in the treatment of muscle tension dysphonia. *Current Opinion in Otolaryngology and Head and Neck Surgery*. *19*:171–6.

Mathieson L (2001) *Greene and Mathieson's the Voice and Its Disorders* (6th edn) London: Whurr Publishers.

Mathieson L, Hirani SP, Epstein R et al. (2009) Laryngeal manual therapy: a preliminary study to examine its treatment effects in the management of muscle tension dysphonia *Journal of Voice* **23**:353–366.

Mathur R, Vishwakarma C, Sinha V et al. (2015) Efficacy of voice therapy in teachers: using perceptual assessment protocol. *Indian Journal of Otology* **21**(2): 149–153.

McCullough GH, Zraick RI, Balou et al. (2012) Treatment of laryngeal hyperfunction with flow phonation: a pilot study *Journal of Laryngology and Voice* **2**: 64–69.

Morsomme D, Faurichon de la Bardonnie M, Verduykt I et al. (2010) Subjective evaluation of the long-term efficacy of speech therapy on dysfunctional dysphonia *Journal of Voice* **24**(2): 178–182.

Nemr K, Simoes-Zenari M, Ferro Cordeiro G et al. (2012) GRBAS and CAPE-V scales: high reliability and consensus when applied at different times. *Journal of Voice* **26**(6): 812–817.

Nguyen DD, Kenny DT (2009) Randomized controlled trial of vocal function exercises on muscle tension dysphonia in Vietnamese female teachers *Journal of Otolaryngology-Head and Neck Surgery* **38**: 261–278.

Niebudek-Bogusz E, Sznurowska-Przygocka B, Fiszer M et al. (2008) The effectiveness of voice therapy of teachers with dysphonia *Folia Phoniatrica et Logopaedica* **60**:134–141.

Oates J (2009) Auditory-perceptual evaluation of disordered voice quality *Folia Phoniatrica et Logopaedica* **61**: 49–56.

Oates J, Winkworth A (2008) Current knowledge, controversies and future directions in hyperfunctional voice disorders *International Journal of Speech-Language Pathology* **10**: 267–277.

Ogawa M, Hosokawa K, Yoshida M et al. (2014) Immediate effects of humming on computed electroglottographic parameters in patients with muscle tension dysphonia *Journal of Voice* **28**(6): 733–741.

Paes SM, Zambon F, Yamasaki R et al. (2013) Immediate effects of the Finnish resonance tube method on behavioural dysphonia *Journal of Voice* **27**(6): 717–722.

Patel RR, Bless DM, Thibeault SL (2011) Boot camp: a novel intensive approach to voice therapy *Journal of Voice* **25**: 562–569.

Pasa G, Oates J, Dacakis G. (2007) The relative effectiveness of vocal hygiene training and vocal function exercises in preventing voice disorders in primary school teachers *Logopedics Phoniatrics Vocology* **32**: 128–140.

Portone-Maira C, Wise JC, Johns MM, Hapner ER (2011) Differences in temporal variables between voice therapy completers and dropouts *Journal of Voice* **25**(1): 62–66.

Rattenbury H, Carding PN, Finn P (2004) Evaluating the effectiveness and efficiency of voice therapy using transnasal flexible laryngoscopy: a randomized controlled trial *Journal of Voice* 18(4): 522–533.

Robey RR (2004) A five-phase model for clinical outcome research *Journal of Communication Disorders* 37: 401–411

Rodriguez-Parra MJ, Adrian JA, Casado JC (2011) *Journal of Communication Disorders* 44: 615–630.

Rosen CA, Lees AS, Osborne J et al. (2004) Development and validation of the Voice Handicap Index-10 *Laryngoscope* 9: 1549–1556.

Roy N (2008) Assessment and treatment of musculoskeletal tension in hyperfunctional voice disorder *International Journal of Speech-Language Pathology* 10: 195–209.

Roy N (2003) Functional dysphonia *Current Opinion in Otolaryngology and Head and Neck Surgery* 11: 144–148.

Roy N, Barkmeier-Kramer J, Eadie T et al. (2012) Evidence-based clinical voice assessment: A systematic review *American Journal of Speech Language Pathology* 22(2): 212–226.

Rubin JS, Blake E, Mathieson L (2007) Musculoskeletal patterns in patients with voice disorders *Journal of Voice* 21(4): 477–484.

Ruotsalainen JH, Sellman J, Lehto L et al. (2009) Interventions for treating functional dysphonia in adults (review) *The Cochrane Library* 3: 1–29.

Sama A, Carding PN, Price S et al. (2001) The clinical features of functional dysphonia *Laryngoscope* 11(3): 458–463.

Schwartz SR, Cohen SM, Dailey S et al (2009) Clinical practice guideline: Hoarseness *Otolaryngology–Head and Neck Surgery* 141(3, Suppl. 2): S1–S31.

Sellars C, Carding P, Deary IJ et al. (2002) Characterization of effective primary voice therapy for dysphonia *The Journal of Laryngology and Otology* 116(12): 1014–1018.

Shewell C (2009) *Voice Work – Art and Science in Changing Voices* Chichester: Wiley-Blackwell.

Simberg S, Laine A (2007) The resonance tube method in voice therapy: description and practical implementations *Logopedics Phoniatrics Vocology* 32: 165–170.

Simberg S, Sala E, Tuomainen J et al. (2006) The effectiveness of group therapy for students with mild voice disorders: a controlled clinical trial *Journal of Voice* 20(1): 97–109.

Smith BE, Kempster GB, Sims HS (2010) Patient factors related to voice therapy attendance and outcomes *Journal of Voice* 24(6): 694–701.

Solomon NP (2008) Vocal fatigue and its relation to vocal hyperfunction *International Journal of Speech-Language Pathology* 10: 254–266.

Speyer R (2008) Effects of voice therapy: a systematic review *Journal of Voice* 22: 565–580.

Speyer R, Wieneke GH, Dejonckere PH (2004) Documentation in progress in voice therapy: Perceptual, acoustic and laryngostroboscopic findings pretherapy and posttherapy *Journal of Voice* 18: 325–340.

Stemple JC, Glaze L, Klaben B (2010) *Clinical Voice Pathology: Theory and Management* (4th edn) San Diego, CA: Plural Publishing, Inc.

Stepp CE, Sawin DE, Eadie TL (2012) The relationship between perception of vocal effort and relative fundamental frequency during voicing offset and onset *Journal of Speech, Language and Hearing Research* 55: 1887–1896.

Stepp CE, Merchant GR, Heaton JT, Hillman RE (2011) Effects of voice therapy on relative fundamental frequency during voicing offset and onset in patients with vocal hyperfunction *Journal of Speech, Language and Hearing Research* 54: 1260–1266.

Story BH, Laukkanen A, Titze IR (2000) Acoustic impedance of an artificially lengthened and constricted vocal tract *Journal of Voice* 14(4): 455–469.

Taylor-Goh S (Ed.) (2005) *RCSLT Clinical Guidelines* Bicester: Speechmark.

Thyme-Frokjaer K, Frokjaer-Jensen B (2001) *The Accent Method - A Rational Voice Therapy in Theory and Practice* Bicester: Speechmark.

Titze IR (2006) Voice training and therapy with a semi-occluded vocal tract: rationale and scientific underpinnings *Journal of Speech, Language and Hearing Research* 49: 448–459.

Titze IR, Verdolini Abbott K (2013) *Vocology: The Science and Practice of Voice Rehabilitation* Oxford: Compton Publishing.

Tomlinson CA, Archer KR (2015) Manual therapy and exercise to improve outcome in patients with muscle tension dysphonia *Physical Therapy* 95: 117–128.

Van Houtte E, Van Lierde K, D'Haeseleer E *et al.* (2009) The prevalence of laryngeal pathology in a treatment-seeking population with dysphonia *Laryngoscope* 120: 306–312.

Van Houtte E, Claeys S, D'haeseleer E *et al.* (2013) An examination of surface EMG for the assessment of muscle tension dysphonia *Journal of Voice* 27: 177–186.

Van Leer E, Connor NP (2011) Use of portable media players increases patient motivation and practice in voice therapy *Journal of Voice* 26(4): 447–453.

Van Leer E, Connor NP (2010) Patient perceptions of voice therapy adherence *Journal of Voice* 24(4): 458–469.

Van Lierde KM, De Bodt M, Dhaeselaer E *et al.* (2010) The treatment of muscle tension dysphonia: a comparison of two treatment techniques by means of an objective multiparameter approach *Journal of Voice* 24: 294–301.

Van Lierde KM, Claes S, De Bodt M, Van Cauwenberge P (2007) Long-term outcome of hyperfunctional voice disorders based on a multi-parameter approach *Journal of Voice* 21(2): 179–188.

Verdolini Abbott K (2008) *Lessac-Madsen Resonant Voice Therapy*. San Diego, CA: Plural Publishing, Inc.

Voerman MS, Langeveld APM, van Rossum MA (2008) Retrospective study of 116 patients with non-organic voice disorders: efficacy of mental imagery and laryngeal shaking *Journal of Laryngology and Otology* 123: 528-34.

Voigt D, Dollinger M, Braunschweig T *et al.* (2010) Classification of functional voice disorders based on phonovibrograms *Artificial Intelligence in Medicine* 49(1): 51–59.

Watts CR, Diviney SS, Hamilton A *et al.* (2014) The effects of stretch and flow voice therapy on measures of vocal function and handicap *Journal of Voice* 29(2): 191–199.

Welham NV (2009) Clinical voice evaluation In: AE Aronson and DM Bless (Eds.) *Clinical Voice Disorders* (4th edn) New York, NY: Thieme, pp134–165.

Wenke RJ, Stabler P, Walton C *et al.* (2014) Is more intensive better? Client and service provider outcomes for intensive versus standard therapy schedules for functional dysphonia *Journal of Voice* 28(5): 652–666.

Wilson J, Deary I, Millar A, (2002) The quality of life impact of functional dysphonia *Clinical Otolaryngology* 27: 179–182.

Ziegler A, Dastolfo C, Hersan R *et al.* (2014) Perceptions of voice therapy form patients diagnosed with primary muscle tension dysphonia and benign mid-membranous vocal fold lesions *Journal of Voice* 28(6): 742–752.

Ziegler A, Gillespie AI, Verdolini-Abbott K (2010) Behavioural treatment of voice disorders in teachers *Folia Phoniatrica et Logopaedica* 62(1–2): 9–23.

# 4

# The effectiveness of voice therapy for vocal fold nodules

## Sherry Fu and Paul Carding

## Introduction

Vocal fold nodules are common, benign, laryngeal pathologies and their presence can result in significant voice deterioration (Colton, *et al.*, 2006; Kunduk and McWhorter, 2009; Pannbacker, 1999). They are believed to be caused by repetitive mucosal injury leading to histological changes and concomitant voice changes (Kent and Ball, 2000). They are generally localised masses, bilateral although not always symmetrical and located within the lamina propria typically at the midpoint of the membranous vocal folds (i.e., at the junction of the anterior third and posterior two thirds of the full length of the vocal fold) (Verdolini *et al.*, 2006). The lesions interfere with the vibratory behaviour of the vocal folds, creating increased aperiodicity which results in symptoms of mild to moderate dysphonia characterised by hoarseness, breathiness, low pitch and laryngeal hyperfunction; hoarseness is the most common symptom (Pannbacker, 1999; Verdolini *et al.*, 2006).

Incidence of vocal nodules appears to be related to occupations involving high voice use, excessive work hours and time spent in the occupation (Fritzell, 1996; Goldman *et al.*, 1996; Holmberg *et al*, 2003; Martins *et al.*, 2010). There is evidence of an increased incidence of vocal fold nodules in, for example, teachers, singers, lawyers, salespeople, preachers and telemarketers (Pannbacker, 1999). Vocal nodules occur more frequently in women than in men, possibly due to hormone-mediated effects (Chodara, *et al*, 2012; Colton *et al.*, 2006; Dejonkere,

2001). A range of personality traits, psychosocial factors and somatic status have been associated with vocal fold nodules (Goldman *et al.*, 1996; Karkos and McCormick, 2009; Roy *et al.*, 2000). Nodules are also frequently observed in individuals with velopharyngeal dysfunction and hearing loss, those who consistently use glottal stop substitutions and children with attention deficit hyperactivity disorder (D'Alatri *et al.*, 2015; Verdolini *et al.*, 2006).

Vocal fold nodules cause voice difficulties that often lead to lost time at work, reduced productivity and impaired quality of life (Kunduk and McWhorter, 2009). The symptoms of dysphonia can adversely affect an individual's professional life. This often leads to disability as voice and speech functions are essential for effective communication, the power of self-assertion and persuasion and hence professional success (Fischer *et al.*, 2009).

## Behavioural voice therapy treatment of vocal fold nodules

### Voice therapy and surgery

Treatment options include either voice therapy from a speech–language pathologist (SLP) only, or a combination of voice therapy and laryngeal microsurgery by an otolaryngologist. However, most authors endorse voice therapy as the primary treatment, with surgery as a secondary alternative should vocal limitations and laryngeal pathology remain after behavioural management (Hogikyan *et al.*, 1999, Sulica and Behrman, 2003). Sataloff (1991) suggested that for longer lasting lesions, voice therapy is the primary treatment and surgery should be reserved for those patients whose dysphonia persisted after 3 to 6 months of intense therapy. However, treatment decisions may also be based on several factors, including age, duration of vocal fold nodules, extent of dysphonia and what treatment options are available (Pannbacker, 1999).

In a recent Cochrane review comparing surgical and non-surgical interventions for vocal fold nodules, the authors found that there is evidence from non-randomised intervention studies that both voice therapy techniques and surgery are effective (Pedersen and McGlashan, 2012). However there is uncertainty as to how patients should be selected for primary voice therapy and which would benefit from surgery. In addition, although voice therapy is a first-line treatment there is no consensus as to which of the techniques used is most effective or how long they should be used. Pedersen and McGlashan (2012) concluded that there is no evidence from randomised controlled trials on which to base reliable conclusions about the comparative effectiveness of surgical versus non-surgical interventions for the management of patients with vocal fold nodules.

## Behavioural voice therapy for vocal fold nodules

Voice therapy is a behavioural intervention that primarily aims to resolve the behavioural component of a voice disorder; it depends inherently on active client involvement (van Leer *et al.*, 2008). Most treatment approaches for vocal fold nodules will include at least three basic components: education of the patient regarding behaviours and practices that produce, maintain and/or exacerbate mid-membranous thickenings; elimination of maladaptive behaviours that result from the vocal fold nodules and further exacerbate pathology; and modification of relevant speaker-specific and situation-specific behaviours implicated in development of the tissue changes (Leonard, 2009). However, in order to reinforce the behavioural change, structured treatment sessions and follow-up practice outside the therapy sessions are required (Portone *et al.*, 2008).

The success rate of voice treatment may depend on factors such as: chronicity, nature of aetiology, medical history, presence or absence of secondary gains, variability of treatment techniques, treatment duration, clinician's skill and knowledge, clinician's personality, client motivation and confidence in treatment, client adherence, client's perception of voice therapy, the need to take time off work to attend therapy and to practice target voice behaviours and the time required to travel to therapy (Patel *et al.*, 2011).

## Effectiveness of voice therapy for vocal fold nodules

A review by Leonard (2009) concluded that voice therapy for vocal nodules can improve tissue health and voice, but complete resolution of pathology may not be possible in all patients, particularly if the basement membrane of the vocal fold cover is permanently altered. Therefore, voice therapy, either independently or in combination with other treatment, is essential in clients with vocal fold nodules. The current literature relating to the efficacy of voice therapy has been summarised in Table 1, which shows that existing studies vary in nature and design and can be classified as predominantly Phase 1 studies. As discussed in Chapter 2, according to Robey (2004), a Phase 1 study aims to detect the presence of a therapeutic effect by using small group, case series or single case studies, while Phase 2 studies refine the population to be studied, define the treatment protocol and determine the most appropriate assessments. By contrast, a Phase 3 study is carried out to provide stronger evidence of treatment efficacy, using large sample sizes and parallel groups design. A Phase 4 study determines whether the treatment effects observed in efficacy studies also translate into a clinical environment and a Phase 5 study tests the cost-effectiveness of the

Table 1: Studies of Voice Treatment for Vocal Fold Nodules

| Authors | Number of participants | Type of treatment | Duration and intensity of treatment | Outcome measures | Findings |
|---|---|---|---|---|---|
| **Phase 1 studies (Robey 2004)** | | | | | |
| Fisher and Logemann (1970) | 1 Woman | Habituation of higher pitch | Unspecified | Laryngoscopy ratings | 1. Marked reduction in size of vocal fold nodules. 2. Marked reduction in the speed quotient accompanied with elevation of pitch. 3. Increased open quotient both in the posterior glottis and the anterior glottis. (No statistical analysis available) |
| Drudge and Philips (1976) | 3 College students | 31-step voice therapy programme | 8 weeks; 16 half-hour sessions | Percentages of correct responses | All students demonstrated improvements in behavioural responses after therapy. (No statistical analysis available) |
| Hufnagle and Hufnagle (1984) | 8 Women | Voice modification programme | Unspecified | 1. Voice quality ratings 2. Speaking $F_0$ measurements | 1. Speaking $F_0$ – no significant differences ($p > 0.01$) 2. Some changes in voice quality ratings (no statistical analysis available). |
| McFarlane and Watterson (1990) | 44 Patients (11 children, 33 adults) | Voice therapy (vocal hygiene, abuse reduction and vocal retraining) | Ranging from five to fifty 30-minute sessions Twice weekly | 1. Acoustic measures 2. Laryngoscopy ratings | 1. Voice normalises and vocal fold nodules are completely eliminated. 2. No scarring of vocal folds after therapy and nodules do not return. 3. Less than 1% of patients have return of nodules 1 year later. (No statistical analysis available) |

| Authors | Number of participants | Type of treatment | Duration and intensity of treatment | Outcome measures | Findings |
|---|---|---|---|---|---|
| Murry and Woodson (1992) | 59 Adults (48 women, 11 men) | Group 1: voice therapy Group 2: surgery followed by voice therapy; Group 3: voice therapy + endoscopy | Average number of visits: Group 1 = not reported Group 2 = 11.2 Group 3 = 7.5 Unspecified intensity | 1. Voice quality ratings 2. Laryngoscopy ratings | 1. Group 3 had the highest overall improvement (no statistical analysis available). 2. Group 3 required the least number of visits. 3. Groups 1 and 2 demonstrated improvement in the post-treatment condition, but less than that of group 3 (no statistical analysis available). 4. Mean differences between groups 1 and 2 and between groups 2 and 3 were significant ($p < 0.05$). |
| Schneider (1993) | 1 Woman | Vocal hygiene counselling | 12 weeks; seven assessments over two years. One session/week | 1. Voice quality rating 2. Laryngoscopy 3. Acoustic measures 4. Patient rating of own voice | 1. Voice quality judgements tended to relate to the changes in degree of vocal fold pathology and patient report of vocal function. 2. Significant improvement in voice was reported by patients post-treatment. 3. No vocal fold nodules were visible at the end of the seventh visit. (No statistical analysis available) |
| Blood (1994) | 2 Women | Computer-assisted voice treatment; relaxation | 17–21 sessions. Unspecified intensity | 1. Voice quality ratings 2. Acoustic measures 3. Laryngoscopy ratings | 1. Voice treatment resulted in improved voice quality, elimination of nodules, ratings of clients and social validation measures. 2. Relaxation component used was not associated with clinically significant improvements in patients' voices. (No statistical analysis available) |

| Authors | Number of participants | Type of treatment | Duration and intensity of treatment | Outcome measures | Findings |
|---|---|---|---|---|---|
| Verdolini-Marston et al., (1994) | 6 Women with vocal fold nodules or polyps | Double-blind: hydration treatment and placebo/control treatment | Two sets of five consecutive days over two weeks Daily (intensive) | 1. Voice quality ratings 2. Acoustic measures 3. Laryngoscopy | 1. Significantly overall superior hydration effect when compared with placebo/control treatment ($p < 0.05$) 2. Perceived phonatory effort: significant improvements with hydration treatment but not with the placebo/control treatment (no statistical analysis available). 3. Larynges appeared the best following the hydration treatment for majority of subjects (no statistical analysis available). 4. Average jitter, shimmer and signal to noise ratio improved somewhat following the placebo/control treatment and they were best following the hydration treatment (no statistical analysis available) |
| Verdolini-Marston et al., (1995) | 13 Women | Confidential vs resonant voice therapy | Nine sessions over 12 days, 1 hour sessions | 1. Auditory perceptual ratings 2. Phonatory effect ratings 3. Visual perceptual ratings 4. Client impression | 1. With both types of therapy (confidential vs resonant voice therapy), a greater proportion of therapy subjects showed improvements in all measures (phonatory effort, auditory-perceptual and visual-perceptual) over the initial 2-week period, as compared with control subjects (no statistical analysis available). 2. No identifiable relationship between the type of therapy that was administered and the likelihood of benefiting from therapy ($p > 0.05$ on all measures) |

| Authors | Number of participants | Type of treatment | Duration and intensity of treatment | Outcome measures | Findings |
|---|---|---|---|---|---|
| Lockhart et al., (1997) | 25 Adults | Unspecified type of voice therapy | From two to 16 sessions. Unspecified intensity | 1. Aerodynamic measurement 2. EGG 3. Pitch range 4. Stroboscopy ratings | Improvements in vital capacity, mean/peak airflow ratio, % voicing time in reading, as well as the EGG results of closure time and opening fraction. (No statistical analysis available) |
| Treole and Trudeau (1997) | 13 Women | Tension identification, vocal abuse identification and elimination, laryngeal strengthening | From six to 26 sessions. Unspecified intensity | 1. MPT of notes and vowels 2. s/z ratio | Did not demonstrate change over course of treatment ($p > 0.05$ on all measures). |
| Trullinger et al., (1998) | 1 Woman | Relaxation, vocal hygiene | Three weeks. Unspecified intensity | 1. Voice quality ratings 2. Acoustic analysis 3. Laryngoscopy | 1. Perceived voice quality improved (no statistical analysis available). 2. Reduction in vowel SNL ($p < 0.05$). 3. Increase in vowel $F_0$ (no statistical analysis available). 4. Reduction in vocal fold nodules (no statistical analysis available). |

| Authors | Number of participants | Type of treatment | Duration and intensity of treatment | Outcome measures | Findings |
|---|---|---|---|---|---|
| Holmberg et al., (2001) | 11 Women | Five phases: vocal hygiene, direct facilitation, respiration, relaxation, carryover | From 4–6 months One session/week. Three sessions of each approach | 1. Voice quality ratings<br>2. Acoustic analysis<br>3. Laryngoscopy ratings | 1. Nodules did not disappear but did decrease in size for 9 clients (no statistical analysis available).<br>2. No significant change in SPL (loudness), increased significantly in $F_0$ ($p < 0.05$).<br>3. Significant effects of therapy were found for decreased values of press, instability gratings, roughness, vocal fry, scrape and overall dysphonia ($p < 0.05$). |
| Holmberg et al., (2003) | 10 Women | Five phases: vocal hygiene, direct facilitation, respiration, relaxation and carry over | Varied between 4 and 6 months One session/week | 1. Laryngeal examination<br>2. Aerodynamic measures<br>3. Acoustic measures | 1. Laryngoscopic ratings improvements (but nodules not completely resolved) (no statistical analysis available).<br>2. Neither the acoustic nor the aerodynamic parameters changed significantly across the voice therapy ($p > 0.05$). |
| van der Merwe (2004) | 1 Woman with bilateral vocal fold nodules (case study)<br>10 Adults with nodules (questionnaire on value of programme) | Voice use reduction programme | 10 weeks One session/week | 1. Laryngoscopy<br>2. Voice quality ratings<br>3. Acoustic voice analyses | 1. Nodules were no longer visible after 6 weeks of the programme.<br>2. Acoustic parameters had improved or were within the normal range after 2 weeks into the programme.<br>3. Perceptual voice quality improved.<br>(No statistical analysis available) |

| Authors | Number of participants | Type of treatment | Duration and intensity of treatment | Outcome measures | Findings |
|---|---|---|---|---|---|
| Chernobelsky (2007) | 1 Male and 27 Women | Ultrasound therapy and singing lessons combined | From 3–4 months Unspecified intensity | 1. Acoustic measures 2. Laryngoscopy ratings | 1. No differences in speaking $F_0$ pre- and post-therapy ($p > 0.05$). 2. Decreased jitter and shimmer values and increase of signal noise ratio post-therapy ($p < 0.05$). 3. Reoccurrence of vocal fold nodules common. |
| Fu et al., (2015b) | 10 Women | Intensive voice therapy delivered via telepractice | 3 weeks; 9 sessions of 45 minutes each. Intensive: 3 times a week | 1. Voice quality ratings 2. Stroboscopic ratings 3. Aerodynamic measures 4. Acoustic measures 5. VHI | 1. Significantly improved ratings on perceptual parameters of voice quality ($p < 0.05$). 2. Stroboscopic rating improvements in mucosal wave, vocal fold smoothness and glottal closure ($p < 0.05$). 3. Positive changes in acoustic parameters ($p < 0.05$) 4. Significant increase in mean airflow rate ($p < 0.05$) 5. Total VHI score decreased significantly post therapy ($p < 0.05$). |
| **Phase 2 studies (Robey 2004)** | | | | | |
| Niebudek-Bogusz et al., (2008a) | 46 Female teachers with functional voice disorders (incuding vocal fold nodules) | Vocal training (group 1) and vocal hygiene (group 2) | Over 3 months, each session lasting for 45 minutes One session/week | 1. VHI 2. Laryngoscopy 3. Acoustic analyses 4. Aerodynamic measures (MPT) | 1. MPT increased significantly in group 1 ($p < 0.05$), but not in group 2 ($p > 0.05$). 2. Videostroboscopic parameters (amplitude and mucosal wave) revealed significant post-therapy improvement in group 1 ($p < 0.05$). 3. Significant increase in the mean $F_0$ noted in group 1 only (no statistical analysis available). 4. Other acoustic parameters (jitter, RAP, PPQ) of both groups were improved post-treatment, especially group 1 ($p < 0.05$). |

| Authors | Number of participants | Type of treatment | Duration and intensity of treatment | Outcome measures | Findings |
|---|---|---|---|---|---|
| Niebudek-Bogusz et al., (2008b) | 186 Female teachers (including vocal nodules) | Voice trained group and non-voice-trained group | Ranging from 2 to 4 months, each session lasting for 45 to 60 minutes Once to twice/week | 1. Stroboscopy ratings 2. Aerodynamic measures MPT 3. Acoustic analysis | 1. Videostroboscopic parameters improved with voice-trained group only ($p < 0.05$). 2. Voice quality parameters improved with voice-trained group only ($p < 0.05$). 3. MPT ($p < 0.05$), mean $F_0$ ($p > 0.05$), mean vocal intensity ($p > 0.05$) and voice frequency range ($p < 0.05$) were increased in voice-trained group only. |
| Phase 3 studies (Robey 2004) | | | | | |
| Sellars et al., (2002) | 204 Participants with either functional dysphonia, mild laryngitis, small nodules or muscle tension dysphonia | Randomly allocated: treatment group or control group | Maximum of six sessions, 50 minutes/session Unspecified intensity | 1. Carding Vocal Performance Questionnaire 2. Buffalo III Voice Profile 3. Voice measures | 1. Significant improvement in voice quality following a general programme of voice therapy relying heavily on indirect therapy strategies (no statistical analysis available). 2. Significant benefits in both the VPQ ($p < 0.05$) and the Buffalo scale ($p < 0.05$) |
| Fu et al., (2015a) | 53 Women | Intensive group and traditional group | one session of vocal hygiene and 8 sessions of direct treatment, 45 minutes/session Intensive group: 2–3 sessions/week Traditional group: 1 session/week | 3. Voice quality ratings 4. Stroboscopy ratings 5. Acoustic analysis 6. Aerodynamic analysis | 1. Significant improvements for both groups for stroboscopic ratings ($p < 0.05$). 2. Significant increase in $F_0$ and significant reduction in jitter and shimmer were found in both groups post treatment ($p < 0.05$). 3. No significant differences were found between groups in all investigated measures ($p > 0.05$). |

| Authors | Number of participants | Type of treatment | Duration and intensity of treatment | Outcome measures | Findings |
|---|---|---|---|---|---|
| Fu et al., (2016) | 36 Women | Intensive group and traditional group | One session of vocal hygiene and 8 sessions of direct treatment, 45 minutes/session Intensive group: 2–3 sessions/week Traditional group: 1 session/week | 1. Voice quality ratings 2. Stroboscopy ratings 3. Acoustic analysis 4. VHI | 1. Both TVT and IVT groups had significantly improved voice quality ratings ($p < 0.05$). 2. By 6 months post-treatment both groups continued to present with improvements in voice quality ratings ($p < 0.05$). 3. Both groups had significant improvements in stroboscopy ratings ($p < 0.05$). (post-treatment and at 6 month follow-up). 4. Both groups had significantly reduced vocal nodule size at 6 month follow-up ($p < 0.05$). 5. Significant increases in $F_0$ in both groups at both post-treatment and 6 months ($p < 0.05$). 6. Only IVT group showed improvements in jitter, shimmer, NHR and vocal intensity of prolonged vowel at 6 months compared to baseline ($p < 0.05$). 7. Both groups had significant changes in total VHI score post-treatment which was maintained at 6 months post-treatment ($p < 0.05$). |

Note. VHE = vocal hygiene education; VP = voice production; $F_0$ = fundamental frequency; PTP = phonation threshold pressure; VI = vocal intensity; MPT = maximum phonation time; RAP = relative average perturbation; PPQ = pitch perturbation quotient; SLP = Speech-Language Pathologist; SPL = speech pressure level; EGG = electroglottography; VPQ = Carding Vocal Performance Questionnaire; VHI = Voice Handicap Index; SNL = spectral noise level; TVT = traditional voice therapy; IVT = intensive voice therapy.

treatment and assesses consumer satisfaction and broader issues pertaining to the social and political environment of health service delivery, including the worth of a treatment. Currently, within the available research articles for vocal fold nodules there is a paucity of Phase 2–5 studies.

## Phase 1 efficacy studies

Several Phase 1 studies including single case and small group studies (without control group comparison) have reported perceptual, physiological and acoustic improvements post-voice treatment using various combinations of therapy techniques (Drudge and Philips, 1976; Fisher and Logemann, 1970; Holmberg *et al.*, 2001; Holmberg *et al.*, 2003; Schneider, 1993; Trullinger, *et al.*, 1988).

All the single case studies (Fisher and Logemann, 1970; Schneider 1993; Trullinger *et al*, 1998) showed marked improvements in voice quality, vocal nodule appearance and/or self-report. In Schneider's single case study, the participant received 12 sessions of vocal hygiene counselling, provided once weekly. The participant reported significant improvement in voice production following five sessions of voice therapy, with her vocal range returning by the sixth session of voice therapy to what it was prior to the three-year period of dysphonia. The self-report correlated with the improved voice quality ratings by the SLPs and the laryngologist's finding that the vocal fold nodules were no longer visible at the final session. However, no acoustic changes were observed. These results were similar to those reported by Trullinger *et al.*, (1998) in a case study of an individual with bilateral vocal fold nodules who underwent three weeks of voice therapy. It was found that after treatment, only slight erythema of the true vocal folds remained and there was improvement in perceived voice quality as well as a measured reduction in vowel spectral noise level. In addition, the participant had an increase in vowel $F_0$. The participant was able to maintain these improvements for an extended time following discharge from therapy. Drudge and Philips (1976) reported on a case series of three participants with vocal fold nodules using a 31-step voice therapy programme. They demonstrated that in two of the participants the nodules had been eliminated and the third showed a reduction of the nodule formation post-intervention. Although this study reported that the therapy programme took a total of 16 sessions over an 8-week period, the distribution of the sessions was not documented.

In addition to single case and case series data, many of the studies to date have conducted small group cohort studies. Hufnagle and Hufnagle (1984) investigated the relationship between improved vocal quality and speaking $F_0$

in eight women with vocal fold nodules following voice therapy. It was found there were no significant differences between the before and after speaking $F_0$, although the listeners who rated the voice "preferred" the vocal quality following therapy. Holmberg et al., (2001) examined the efficacy of a behaviourally-based voice therapy programme for vocal fold nodules in 11 women, provided on a once-weekly basis. The voice therapy consisted of five basic phases: vocal hygiene, direct facilitation, respiration, relaxation and carryover. The total therapy period varied between four and six months, depending on the attendance of the clients. Overall, dysphonia was found to have decreased significantly after therapy. However, although almost all of the participants' vocal fold nodules had decreased in size, none of them had resolved after completion of the therapy. The outcome suggested that the voice therapy had a positive effect for a majority of patients (Holmberg et al., 2001). Similar results were yielded in a later study by Holmberg et al., (2003) involving 10 women with bilateral vocal fold nodules. The same voice therapy techniques were used for four to six months and were also provided on a weekly basis. Laryngoscopic examinations showed that the vocal fold nodules had decreased in size and surrounding oedema had dissipated, after completion of voice therapy, suggesting that the trauma to the vocal folds had indeed decreased after the therapy. However, it was found that the improved vocal fold appearances were not reflected in the acquired aerodynamic and acoustic measures. Unlike other small group studies, none of the participants had resolved nodules.

In a larger group study of 25 participants with vocal fold nodules Lockhart et al., (1997) demonstrated that after voice therapy, participants had improvement in the vital capacity, mean/peak airflow ratio and percentage voicing time in reading, as well as in the electroglottography results. The therapy sessions provided for this study ranged from 2 to 16 with treatment duration ranging from 16 to 24 weeks. The study provided some indication of the length of treatment for different degrees of severity (i.e., larger vocal fold nodules required a longer care period). McFarlane and Watterson (1990) also reported success in 44 individuals with vocal fold nodules. Their voice therapy ranged from five to 50 sessions (30 minutes twice weekly). The vocal fold nodules were reported to have completely resolved after voice treatment using a combination of vocal hygiene, vocal abuse reduction and vocal re-education. Less than 1% of their patients had experienced a return of nodules one year later. The authors reported nodular recurrence in only one patient.

The support for behavioural treatment has also been noted in surveys and in retrospective studies (Hogikyan et al., 1999; Lancer et al., 1988; Murry and Woodson, 1992). A questionnaire survey showed that the majority of professionals involved in the care of singers with vocal fold nodules prefer voice therapy alone provided by SLPs and not voice training alone provided by teachers of singing (Hogikyan *et al.*, 1999). In addition, the majority of the surveys show that surgery is appropriate only if behavioural management fails. Therefore, coordinated voice therapy and voice training would be considered as first line treatment. Despite the valuable insights into the opinions of professionals with regard to the treatment of singers with vocal fold nodules, the study did not represent outcomes research (Hogikyan *et al.*, 1999).

Lancer *et al.*, (1988) conducted a retrospective study on 34 participants diagnosed as having either unilateral or bilateral vocal fold nodules. The authors compared the results of three management programmes for vocal fold nodules: surgery, voice therapy, or a combination of the two. It was found that voice treatment (with or without surgery) reduced the incidence of recurrence of vocal fold nodules. No recurrence was diagnosed in participants who had speech therapy, either alone or with surgery. Murry and Woodson (1992) reached similar conclusions following their study of 59 participants with vocal fold nodules. They found that participants who were treated with an integrated approach involving both an SLP and an otolaryngologist demonstrated greater improvement than those who underwent therapy after surgery and those who underwent therapy alone.

## Phase 2 efficacy studies

The positive findings of the majority of the Phase 1 studies are supported by Phase 2 studies which have investigated the efficacy of various forms of voice treatment using a range of group comparison designs. These studies do not specifically examine patients with vocal nodules but include them in larger groups with "functional voice disorders" (or similar terms). It is not possible to extrapolate data on the vocal nodules patients from the broader dataset. The effect of receiving vocal hygiene instructions with additional vocal training, versus vocal hygiene instruction alone, was examined in 46 female teachers with a functional voice disorder including vocal fold nodules, glottal insufficiency, hyperfunction dysphonia (Niebudek-Bogusz *et al.*, 2008a). Thirty participants received both vocal training and vocal hygiene instructions and the remaining 16 received only vocal hygiene instructions. The voice training sessions were conducted once a week, 45 minutes each session and lasted for an average of three months. It was found that those who underwent additional vocal training gained statistically significant improvement in maximum phonation time and $F_0$, whilst no changes were observed for those who underwent vocal hygiene sessions only. Niebudek-Bogusz et al., (2008a) interpreted the significant increase in $F_0$ as a sign of voice quality improvement. Laryngo-videostroscopic parameter ratings also revealed statistically significant post-therapy improvement in the group with additional vocal training. Other acoustic parameters such as jitter, relative average perturbation and amplitude perturbation quotient were found to have improved in both treatment groups. In addition, the authors reported a good correlation between the perceptual and instrumental measures. The authors concluded that the voice stability improvement may be the effect of vocal training. Hence, vocal training may play a role in protecting the laryngeal organ against undesirable changes related to vocal loading for professional voice users.

In a larger group study, Niebudek-Bogusz et al., (2008b) examined the effectiveness of voice therapy on 186 female teachers with hyperfunctional dysphonia, including those with "secondary" chronic laryngitis, vocal fold nodules and minor polypoid hypertrophy. The participants were also divided into two groups: a voice-trained group and a non-voice-trained group. Both groups received advice on vocal hygiene. The vocal training programme comprised breathing and relaxation exercises, vocal function exercises, resonant improvement exercises and carryover exercises. The duration of the voice training varied from two to four months and the number of sessions ranged from nine to 18; each session lasted for 45 to 60 minutes and was given once or twice a week. The results indicated that the voice-trained teachers showed improved voice quality whereas the non-voice-trained teachers showed no improvements based on the following parameters: maximum phonation time, mean $F_0$, voice intensity and voice frequency range during speaking. There was no report of statistical analysis between the two groups in any of the measures investigated.

## Phase 3 efficacy studies

Further to these Phase 1 and Phase 2 efficacy studies, a higher evidence study (Phase 3 – Robey 2004) has also been conducted which confirmed the benefits of voice therapy for vocal fold nodules. Sellars et al., (2002) conducted a randomised controlled trial (RCT) with 204 participants who presented with functional dysphonia, mild laryngitis, small vocal nodules or muscle tension dysphonia. Patients were randomly allocated to a voice treatment group or a control group. However, they were not blind to the type of treatment received. The treatment group received a maximum of six sessions, with each session lasting around 50 minutes. A statistically significant improvement was observed in voice quality following general voice therapy which relied heavily on indirect strategies. This study further confirmed the effectiveness of voice therapy when treating patients with dysphonia, including those with vocal fold nodules. However, specific evidence of the treatment effectiveness of patients with vocal nodules cannot be determined from the data presented in this study.

A recent study investigated the optimal intensity of voice therapy for individuals with vocal fold nodules. Fu and *et al.*, (2015a) examined the effectiveness of intensive voice therapy (eight sessions delivered over three weeks) versus traditional weekly voice therapy (eight sessions delivered over eight weeks) in a group of 53 women with vocal fold nodules. Statistically significant improvements were found in the vocal qualities of both groups, consistent with the physiological findings that there were significant reductions in nodule size and surrounding oedema. The results of the acoustic analyses also revealed that there were significant increases in $F_0$ and decreases in jitter and shimmer, immediately after voice treatment in both groups. Overall, this investigation showed that both treatment approaches could improve vocal fold condition and vocal function. The authors also demonstrated that participants were able to improve voice and vocal fold health much more quickly with the intensive therapy approach and therefore, the intensive model may be more time efficient and beneficial for professional voice users (Fu *et al.*, 2015a).

## Long term benefits of therapy

As shown in the sections above, there is a relatively large body of evidence which has demonstrated, through various types of study design, that there is a positive treatment effect post-behavioural therapy for vocal fold nodules. However, the vast majority of these have only reported the immediate benefits of treatment. As incorrect voice use and vocally-damaging behaviour are often the primary causes of vocal fold nodules, it is crucial that therapy leads to long-term changes in voice use to help prevent nodules from re-occurring.

Two retrospective studies provide early evidence for the long-term benefit of voice therapy. Koufman and Blalock (1989) conducted a retrospective study over a 10-year period on 127 patients with various vocal fold lesions, including vocal fold nodules. They found that for patients with vocal fold nodules, behavioural modification through patient education provided the principal long-term therapeutic benefit. Without such changes in motivation and subsequent behaviour, vocal nodules are likely to recur (Koufman and Blalock, 1989). Lancer *et al.*, (1988) also conducted a retrospective long-term follow-up on patients who have received voice therapy with or without surgery and patients who were treated by surgery alone. They reported that three to five years after the end of treatment, those who received voice therapy with or without surgery had a reduced incidence of recurrence.

Studies which examined outcomes at three months post-therapy also found that short-term benefits were maintained (Blood, 1994; Speyer *et al.*, 2003) and Blood (1993) reported that the benefits of the dependent variables they investigated, including F0, perturbation factor percentage, production of easy onset of air volume, level of tension and stress and self-perception of voice, were maintained over a three-month follow-up. It was further demonstrated by Speyer *et al.*, (2003) that there were still significant changes three months after completion of therapy in the voice range profile, characterised by increased improvement at higher frequencies and intensities. In a recent study, Wenke *et al.*, (2014) compared intensive versus traditional voice therapy in the treatment of clients with functional dysphonia, including vocal fold nodules. The authors found that the intensive group showed a greater improvement at the four weeks follow-up compared with the traditional therapy group. In another recent study, Fu *et al.*, (2016) examined the long-term benefits of intensive voice therapy when compared with traditional voice therapy for patients with vocal fold nodules. They demonstrated that both groups were able to maintain improvements in voice quality and vocal function at six months post-treatment with no significant differences between the groups with respect to degree of changes pre- to 6 months post-treatment and immediately post-treatment to six months post-treatment. Additionally, participants from both groups maintained their self-perception of voice at six months follow-up with no significant differences between the two groups.

In order to ensure that behavioural therapy implemented for vocal fold nodules achieves maintenance of treatment effects beyond the immediate post-treatment period is an area that requires further exploration. To assist clinicians in selecting optimal treatment models for their patients, it is essential that both immediate and long-term outcomes are available for consideration.

## Absence of treatment response

In contrast to the majority of studies which reported success following behavioural voice therapy, a few have failed to demonstrate significant changes in specific parameters following voice therapy. In a retrospective study, Treole and Trudeau (1997) recorded maximum phonation duration for musical notes and vowels and the s/z ratio, to examine differences before and after voice therapy in a group of women with bilateral vocal fold nodules. After therapy, no significant differences were found with the s/z ratio or maximum phonation duration. However, the authors noted that most of the participants began with durational measurements near or within normal limits.

Chernobelsky (2007) carried out a retrospective investigation of the treatment and results of voice therapy amongst 28 professional classical singers with vocal fold nodules. They found no differences in speaking $F_0$ pre- and post-therapy (a predetermined main outcome for this study). However, there was statistically significant decrease in values of magnitudes of jitter and shimmer and a considerable and statistically significant increase in signal-to-noise ratio, which reflected diminishing size of the nodules and indicated a reduction in the vocal noise.

## The range of voice programmes used to manage vocal fold nodules

Even though positive outcomes have been confirmed following voice therapy across a diverse phase of studies, there is a great discrepancy in the components of the therapy programmes administered. In many studies, the actual nature of the tasks and structure of the therapy programme are only briefly and incompletely described. Furthermore, specific information about the intensity (e.g., weekly), duration (length of session) and duration of therapy (weeks, months) are commonly not detailed. As such, it can be problematic for clinicians to implement many of the programmes described into their clinical settings for patients with vocal fold nodules.

### Nature of the therapy programmes

The evidence reported to date shows that a wide range of therapy programmes have been used. Van der Merwe (2004) described a voice use reduction (VUR) programme as part of a holistic treatment approach for clients with small bilateral vocal fold nodules. The treatment involved identification and elimination of vocal hyperfunction, avoidance of high risk factors, the description of problem behaviour in quantitative terms with quantifiable goals set and then application of these self-controls were instructed. The programme passes through three stages (starting with a period of severe voice use reduction and then, as the voice improves, progression to a period of moderate and finally, low voice use reduction), with the duration of each stage reportedly determined by improvement in the condition of the vocal folds, voice quality and/or in the subjective experience of vocal fatigue, vocal effort and laryngeal pain by the client. It was found that after six weeks of moderate VUR and during all follow-up examinations, the participants' vocal fold nodules were no longer visible.

A voice treatment protocol using a computer-assisted biofeedback device was evaluated in two women with bilateral vocal fold nodules by Blood (1994). The biofeedback device was a Computer-Aided Fluency Establishment Trainer (CAFET), consisting of a respiratory sensor, pressure transducer, clip-type microphone and printed circuit board and which plugs into a compatible microcomputer. The software provided coloured computer graphics for visual feedback and functions in real time. Their voice treatment package (12 sessions of treatment) involved seven components: review of anatomy and physiology of laryngeal musculature with normal and pathologic vocal folds voice production and education; identification of misuses and abuses of the voice; establishment of a monitoring programme for abuse and misuse reduction; transfer of the "new voice" to daily living activities; establishment of correct respiratory and supportive breathing habits using CAFET; establishment of easy onset of air volume using CAFET; and relaxation training (Blood, 1994). It was found that the voice treatment was effective in improving the voice, as demonstrated by elimination of the vocal fold nodules, subjective data (ratings of the voice by subjects and naïve listeners) and objective data (changes in $F_0$, maximum phonation time, perturbation factor percentages, breathing errors and slow rise in volume).

Verdolini-Marston et al., (1994) investigated the effect of hydration treatment on six patients with either vocal fold nodules or vocal polyps. The hydration and placebo/control treatment was given on an intensive daily basis (five consecutive days during consecutive weeks). For the hydration treatment, participants were instructed to drink eight or more glasses of water per day and take one teaspoon of a hydration medication (a mucolytic) three times per day at about six-hour intervals; and they were also exposed to high humidity environments in the clinic. For the placebo/control treatment, participants were instructed to perform eight or more sets of 20 bilateral forefinger flexion per day and take one spoon of a herbal medication (actually cherry syrup) three times per day at approximately six-hour intervals; they were exposed to a room with commercial air filters and scented candles for two hours a day in the clinic. In addition to the tasks given, participants had to observe general voice conservation and hygiene measures by limiting heavy voice use, as well as alcohol and caffeine intake and exposure to smoke. General benefits were obtained from both the placebo/control and hydration treatments but overall, significantly greater benefits were obtained from the hydration treatment.

Later, Verdolini-Marston et al., (1995) compared two methods of treatment (confidential voice therapy and resonant voice therapy) on 13 women with vocal fold nodules using measurements of phonatory effort, auditory-perceptual status of voice and laryngeal appearance. Confidential voice therapy involved the production of a minimal intensity, low effort and somewhat breathy phonation mode, similar to speaking confidentially at close quarters. In contrast, resonant voice therapy involved the patients feeling vibratory sensations on the alveolar ridge and other facial plates during phonation, but this approach did not necessarily require quiet voice output. Following two consecutive weeks of intensive treatment (i.e., nine sessions of one hour each over 12 days), both types of voice treatment showed improvements. However, the benefits co-varied directly with estimates of ongoing compliance (extra-clinical utilisation of the therapy technique following therapy discontinuation), but not with therapy type.

## Variability in duration and intensity of treatment

While various voice therapy approaches have been found to be effective for individuals with vocal fold nodules, to date no studies have provided evidence or clear guidelines as to the optimal intensity or duration of voice therapy for this client group. Across the treatment studies conducted, there is considerable variation in the duration of the therapy provided. Some studies on various voice disorders claim significant (short-term) improvement after one single treatment session, whereas others describe the need for a long series of sessions (e.g., four to six months) (Speyer, 2008). It was suggested through a survey by Mueller and Larson (1992) that voice treatment time depends on diagnosis and is usually less than 15 hours (i.e., 6 to 10 hours). Similarly, Colton et al., (2006) suggested that at least six to eight weeks of once a week voice therapy is necessary for improvement in vocal behaviour. In contrast, Verdolini Abbott (2008) suggested that once- to twice-weekly treatment for four to eight weeks is a preferable level of intensity to effect vocal change. Consequently, the optimal intensity of voice therapy for vocal fold nodules remains unresolved.

In some studies of intervention for vocal fold nodules, the number of sessions or duration of voice treatment was reported in days, weeks or years (Pannbacker, 1999). McCrory (2001) stated that in over 90% of clinical records audited, participants required two to 12 sessions of therapy. Lockhart et al., (1988) investigated the time scales for treatment for various laryngeal pathology and they cited a range from two to 16 sessions of voice therapy for vocal fold nodules in the two centres evaluated. A review of the studies of voice therapy for vocal fold nodules showed that the duration of voice treatment varied from 10 consecutive days (Verdolini-Marston et al., 1994) to more than two years (Schneider, 1993), while the intensity of voice treatment varied from daily intensive sessions (Verdolini-Marston et al., 1994; Verdolini-Marston et al., 1995) to the most commonly reported weekly sessions (Behrman et al., 2008; Holmberg et al., 2001; Holmberg et al., 2003; Niebudek-Bogusz et al., 2008b; Niebudek-Bogusz et al., 2008a; Schneider, 1993; van der Merwe, 2004). However, several of the earlier studies provided no information about the duration and intensity of treatment delivered (Fisher and Logeman, 1970; Hufnagle and Hufnagle, 1984; Murry and Woodson, 1992).

As discussed in the previous section, recent research has provided evidence of short-term and long-term benefits for intensive voice therapy (either four 1-hour sessions per week for two weeks, or eight sessions provided over three weeks) for vocal fold nodules and other voice disorders (Fu et al., 2015a, b; Wenke et al., 2014). The reported benefits of intensive voice treatment are as follows: voice improvement can occur in a short period of time; patients' knowledge of tasks for home practice can be enhanced; it is more time efficient for both clinician and client; time between sessions is decreased; the ability to carry over learnt strategies into everyday life is facilitated. Individuals are able to accelerate learning regulated by increasing therapy rate, increasing therapy phase duration, increasing variability of practice and decreasing the rest phase duration (Patel et al, 2011). Intensive contact with the clinician also allows individuals with vocal fold nodules to resolve any queries and be provided with the clinician's feedback regarding use of their voice within a shorter time frame (Fu et al., 2015a). This can help solidify patient awareness and carry-over treatment tasks to daily living (Thibeault et al., 2009). In addition, the intensive treatment schedule may have enhanced motor learning and provided greater opportunity for patients to consolidate vocal hygiene and vocal techniques day-to-day (Wenke et al., 2014). Furthermore, as noted by Spielman et al., (2007), the downfall of prolonged voice therapy extends the time commitment for both client and clinician, with no additional gains to be acknowledged.

## Attendance and adherence data specific to vocal fold nodule therapy

To date, only one study has been published on the individuals with vocal fold nodules adherence to voice treatment, while none has reported on the treatment attendance. Furthermore, no investigation has explored the impact that barriers to access service have on treatment adherence and attendance in individuals with vocal fold nodules. The only study reported to date examined the adherence to instructions regarding general voice hygiene practices and the ongoing adherence following therapy termination, i.e., of the relative continued utilisation of the therapy technique after therapy was discontinued (Verdolini-Marston et al., 1995). The authors found that the participants, regardless of the type of treatment groups, all appeared to follow instructions on general voice hygiene practices to about the same degree. They also indicated that adherence following discontinuation of therapy appeared to be a predictor of longer term improvements in phonatory effort and in auditory perceptual ratings with therapy and is not related to the type of voice therapy received.

## Method of service delivery for vocal fold nodules

Although there is evidence to support the efficacy of voice therapy for vocal fold nodules, access to services remains a potential factor which can limit patients from both seeking and receiving services. To date, the majority of service models examined has focused on therapy delivered via traditional face-to-face (FTF) delivery modes. However, the FTF clinical model may not be possible for many patients because of multiple factors such as inflexible work conditions, absence of locally available services and travel distances. Therefore, there has been increasing interest in the development of alternative models of service delivery for managing patients with vocal fold nodules. One potential solution is the use of telepractice.

Currently, only two investigations have explored the use of telepractice for patients with functional voice disorders, including vocal fold nodules (Fu et al., 2015b; Mashima et al., 2003). In the study conducted by Mashima and colleagues (2003), participants with various functional voice disorders were treated via either conventional therapy or telepractice. The results revealed improvements in voice quality, acoustic and physiological parameters after voice treatment in both the conventional group and telepractice group. The investigators reported that no significant differences were found between groups, indicating that voice therapy delivered remotely was as effective as therapy delivered conventionally

(Mashima et al., 2003). The authors suggested that the use of telepractice would be helpful in overcoming the barrier of geographical distance and eliminating the commute time to the clinics, which interfered with work schedule.

The validity of this mode of service delivery was further supported by a recent study specifically investigating a group of patients with vocal fold nodules. Fu et al., (2015b) explored the possibility of providing intensive voice therapy for vocal fold nodules via telepractice, which may assist with resolving the adherence and attendance issues. Ten participants with bilateral vocal fold nodules were recruited into the study. All participants received one session of vocal hygiene education delivered in FTF format, followed by eight sessions of intensive online voice therapy. The results yielded findings similar to those from their previous study delivered in conventional FTF format (Fu et al., 2015a). Significant improvements were found in perceptual, vocal fold function, acoustic and physiological parameters, and nodule sizes. However, further investigations with larger sample sizes and direct comparison between conventional FTF and telepractice delivery modes are still required to confirm these findings.

# References

Behrman A, Rutledge J, Hembree A, Sheridan S (2008) Vocal hygiene education, voice production therapy and role of patient adherence: A treatment effectiveness study in women with phonotrauma *Journal of Speech, Language and Hearing Research* 51: 350–366.

Blood GW (1994) Efficacy of a computer-assisted voice treatment protocol *American Journal of Speech-Language Pathology* 3: 57–66.

Chernobelsky SI (2007) The treatment and results of voice therapy amongst professional classical singers with vocal fold nodules *Logopedics Phoniatrics Vocology* 32: 178–184.

Chodara AM, Krausert CR, Jiang JJ (2012). Kymographic characterization of vibration in human vocal folds with nodules and polyps *Laryngoscope* 122: 58–65.

Colton RH, Casper JK, Leonard R (2006) *Understanding Voice Problems: A Physiological Perspective for Diagnosis and Treatment* (3rd edn.) Baltimore, MD: Lippincott Williams and Wilkins.

D'Alatri L, Petrelli L, Calò L et al. (2015) Vocal fold nodules in school age children: Attention deficit hyperactivity disorder as a potential risk factor *Journal of Voice* 29 (3): 287–291.

Drudge MK, Philips BJ (1976) Shaping behavior in voice therapy. *Journal of Speech and Hearing Disorders* 41(3): 398–411.

Fischer MJ, Gutenbrunner C, Ptok M (2009) Intensified voice therapy: A new model for the rehabilitation of patients suffering from functional dysphonias *International Journal of Rehabilitation Research* 32(4): 348–355.

Fisher HB, Logemann JA (1970) Objective evaluation of therapy for vocal nodules: A case report *Journal of Speech and Hearing Disorders* **35**: 277–285.

Fritzell B (1996) Voice disorders and occupation *Logopedics Phononiatrics Vocology* **21**: 7–12.

Fu S, Theodoros DG, Ward EC (2015a). Intensive versus traditional voice therapy for vocal nodules: perceptual, physiological, acoustic and aerodynamic changes *Journal of Voice* **29**(2): 260.e31–260.e44.

Fu S, Theodoros DG, Ward EC (2015b). Delivery of intensive voice therapy for vocal fold nodules via telepractice: A pilot feasibility and efficacy study *Journal of Voice* **29**(6) 696–706.

Fu S, Theodoros DG, Ward EC (2016). Long-term effects of an intensive voice treatment for vocal fold nodules. International Journal of Speech-Language, 18 (1), 77–88.

Goldman SL, Hargrave J, Hillman RE *et al.* (1996) Stress, anxiety, somatic complaints and voice use in women with vocal nodules: Preliminary findings. *American Journal of Speech-Language Pathology* **5**: 44–54.

Hogikyan ND, Appel S, Guinn LW, Haxer MJ (1999) Vocal fold nodules in adult singers: Regional opinions about etiologic factors, career impact and treatment. A survey of otolaryngologists, speech pathologists and teachers of singers *Journal of Voice* **13**: 128–142.

Holmberg EB, Doyle P, Perkell JS *et al.* (2003) Aerodynamic and acoustic voice measurements of patients with vocal nodules: Variation in baseline and changes across voice therapy *Journal of Voice* **17**: 262–282.

Holmberg EB, Hillman RE, Hammarberg B *et al* (2001) Efficacy of a behaviorally based voice therapy protocol for vocal nodules *Journal of Voice* **15**: 395–412.

Hufnagle J, Hufnagle K (1984) An investigation of the relationship between speaking fundamental frequency and vocal quality improvement *Journal of Communication Disorders* **17**: 95–100.

Karkos PD, McCormick M (2009) The etiology of vocal fold nodules in adults *Current Opinion in Otolaryngology and Head and Neck Surgery* **17**: 420–423.

Kent RD, Ball MJ (2000) *Voice Quality Measurement* San Diego, CA: Singular.

Koufman JA, Blalock PD (1989) Is voice rest never indicated? *Journal of Voice* **3**(1): 87–91.

Kunduk M, McWhorter AJ (2009) True vocal fold nodules: The role of differential diagnosis *Current Opinion in Otolaryngology and Head and Neck Surgery* **17**: 449–452.

Lancer M, Syder D, Jones AS, Le Boutillier A (1988) The outcome of different management patterns for vocal cord nodules *Journal of Laryngology and Otology* **102**: 423–432.

Leonard R (2009) Voice therapy and vocal nodules in adults *Current Opinion in Otolaryngology and Head and Neck Surgery* **17**: 453–457.

Lockhart MS, Paton F, Pearson L (1997) Targets and timescales: A study of dysphonia using objective assessment *Logopedics Phoniatrics Vocology* **22**: 15–24.

Martins RH, Defaveri J, Custódio Domingues MA *et al.* (2010) Vocal fold nodules: Morphological and immunohistochemical investigations *Journal of Voice* 24(5): 531–539.

Mashima M, Birkmire-Peters D, Syms M *et al.* (2003) Telehealth: Voice therapy using telecommunications technology *American Journal of Speech-Language Pathology* 12: 432–439.

McCrory E (2001) Voice therapy outcomes in vocal fold nodules: a retrospective audit *International Journal of Language and Communication Disorders* 36: 19–24.

McFarlane SC, Watterson TL (1990) Vocal nodules: Endoscopic study of their variations and treatment *Seminars in Speech and Language* 11(1) 47–59.

Murry T, Woodson GE (1992) A comparison of three methods for the management of vocal nodules *Journal of Voice* 6(3): 271–276.

Niebudek-Bogusz E, Kotylo P, Politanski P, Sliwinska-Kowalska M (2008a) Acoustic analysis with vocal loading test in occupational voice disorders: Outcomes before and after voice therapy *International Journal of Occupational Medicine and Environmental Health* 21: 301–308.

Niebudek-Bogusz E, Sznurowska-Przygocka B, Fiszer M *et al.* (2008b) The effectiveness of voice therapy for teachers with dysphonia *Folia Phoniatrica et Logopaedica* 60: 107–162.

Pannbacker M (1999) Treatment of vocal nodules: Options and outcomes *American Journal of Speech-Language Pathology* 8: 209–217.

Patel RR, Bless DM, Thibeault SL (2011) Boot camp: A novel intensive approach to voice therapy *Journal of Voice* 25: 562–569.

Pedersen M, McGlashan J (2012) Surgical versus non-surgical interventions for vocal cord nodules *The Cochrane Database of Systematic Reviews* 13(6): CD001934.

Portone C, Johns MM, Hapner ER (2008) A review of patient adherence to the recommendation for voice therapy *Journal of Voice* 22(2): 192–196.

Robey RR. A five-phase model for clinical outcome research. *Journal of Communication Disorders*. 2004; 37: 401–411

Rosen CA, Gartner-Schmidt J, Hathaway B *et al.* (2012) A nomenclature paradigm for benign midmembranous vocal fold lesions *Laryngoscope* 122: 1335–1341.

Roy N, Bless DM, Heisey D (2000) Personality and voice disorders: A multitrait-multidisorder analysis *Journal of Voice* 14: 521–548.

Sataloff RT (1991) *Professional Voice: The Science and Art of Clinical Care* New York, NY: Raven Press.

Schneider P (1993) Tracking change in dysphonia: a case study *Journal of Voice* 7(2): 179–188.

Sellars C, Carding PN, Deary I *et al* (2002) Characterization of effective primary voice therapy for dysphonia *Journal of Laryngology and Otology* 116: 1014–1018.

Speyer R (2008) Effects of voice therapy: A systematic review *Journal of Voice* 22: 565–580.

Speyer R, Wieneke GH, van Wijck-Warnaar I, Dejonckere PH (2003) Effects of voice therapy on the voice range profile of dysphonic patients *Journal of Voice* 17: 544–556.

Spielman J, Ramig LO, Mahler L *et al.* (2007) Effects of an extended version of the Lee Silverman voice treatment on voice and speech in Parkinson's disease *American Journal of Speech-Language Pathology* **16**: 95–107.

Sulica L, Behrman A (2003). Management of benign vocal fold lesions: A survey of current opinion and practice *Annals of Otology, Rhinology and Laryngology* **112**: 827–833.

Thibeault SL, Zelazny SK, Cohen S (2009) Voice boot camp: Intensive treatment success *The ASHA Leader* **14**: 26–27.

Treole K, Trudeau MD (1997) Changes in sustained production tasks among women with bilateral vocal nodules before and after voice therapy *Journal of Voice* **11**: 462–469.

Trullinger RW, Emanuel FW, Skenes LL, Malpass JC (1988) Spectral noise level measurements used to track voice improvement in one patient *Journal of Communication Disorders* **21**: 447–457.

van der Merwe A (2004) The voice use reduction program *American Journal of Speech-Language Pathology* **13**: 208–218.

van Leer E, Hapner ER, Connor NP (2008) Transtheoretical model of health behavior change applied to voice therapy *Journal of Voice* **22**(6): 688–698.

Verdolini Abbott K (2008) *Lessac-Madsen Resonant Voice Therapy: Clinician Manual*. San Diego, CA: Plural Publishing, Inc.

Verdolini K, Rosen CA, Branski, RC. (2006) *Classification manual of voice disorders – I* Mahwah, NJ: Lawrence Erlbaum Associates.

Verdolini-Marston K, Burke MK, Lessac A *et al.* (1995) Preliminary study of two methods of treatment for laryngeal nodules *Journal of Voice* **9**: 74–85.

Verdolini-Marston K, Sandage M, Titze IR (1994). Effect of hydration treatments on laryngeal nodules and polyps and related voice measures *Journal of Voice* **8**: 30–47.

Wenke RJ, Stabler P, Walton C *et al.* (2014). Is more intensive better? Client and service provider outcomes for intensive versus standard therapy schedules for functional voice disorders *Journal of Voice* **28**(5): 652.e31–652.e43.

# 5

# The effectiveness of voice therapy for mass lesions of the vocal folds

Sue M. Jones and Paul Carding

## Introduction

Vocal fold mass lesions refer to benign growths on the vocal folds which impact upon the vibratory characteristics of the mucosal waveform. Differential diagnosis of these types of lesions can be complex and there is a lack of agreement between clinicians regarding use of a consistent set of terminology (Rosen et al., 2012). These benign laryngeal lesions include vocal nodules, polyps, cysts, pseudocysts and granulomas. However, the evidence for the effectiveness of voice therapy for patients with vocal nodules is considered separately in Chapter 3. Laryngeal polyps, cysts, pseudocysts and granulomas are benign unilateral or bilateral lesions of the vocal folds. These lesions are sometimes associated with other types of vocal fold pathology such as sulcus vocalis, scarring and mucosal bridges (Cornut et al., 1986; Tan and Pitman, 2011). Videolaryngostroboscopy has been show to improve differential diagnosis aiding the choice of appropriate treatments (Colton et al., 1995).

Laryngeal polyps, most commonly found in adults, are located on the free edge of the vocal fold. Appearances can be varied, presenting as round, pedunculated or sessile with a smooth external surface. They may look translucent or, if there has been bleeding, haemorrhagic. Polyps are thought to be caused by acute and/or chronic trauma to the superficial lamina propria resulting in oedema, vessel proliferation and inflammation. Vocal misuse, smoking, gastroesophageal reflux and allergies have all been suggested as possible contributory factors to the development of polyps (Hochman and Zeitels, 2000; Martins *et al.*, 2011a).

Vocal fold cysts are intracordal lesions which can be classified as mucous-retention or epidermic. Both typically give the vocal fold(s) a bulge-like appearance. Cysts can vary in size, sometimes being difficult to detect without the use of videolaryngostroboscopy. Occasionally more than one cyst can be seen with a unilateral vocal fold (Gallivan *et al.*, 2008). Mucous-retention cysts can occur in children but are more commonly seen in adults and are believed to be associated with the obstruction of the glandular ducts. Histology of a mucous-retention cyst shows the presence of mucous within a cavity covered with ciliated cylindrical epithelium. Epidermic cysts occur in the subepithelial layer of the vocal folds and are usually covered in stratified squamous and keratinsed epithelium (Arens *et al.*, 1997; Martins *et al.*, 2011b).

Vocal fold pseudo-cysts have a translucent, blister-like appearance and consist of a semisolid material beneath a thinned epithelium. They are typically more pliable than either polyps or cysts and may have little impact on vocal fold vibration (Estes and Sulica, 2014). Koufman and Belafsky's review of 13 cases of pseudocyst found the occurrence to be most common in women in their fourth decade. A relationship between vocal fold paresis/glottal insufficiency and pseudocysts has also been suggested (Koufman *et al.*, 2001; Rosen *et al.*, 2012).

Vocal fold granulomas, also referred to as contact ulcers, occur on the posterior third (non-vibrating portion) of the vocal fold(s). They may display a smooth or irregular surface: they are usually white in appearance and associated with prolonged intubation, laryngopharyngeal reflux, and hyperfunctional voice characteristics (Martins *et al.*, 2009). Other authors have suggested that granulomas can arise as a result of glottal insufficiency (Carroll *et al.*, 2010). As granulomas occur on the non-vibrating portion of the vocal fold they do not always cause the patient to become dysphonic.

Mass lesions of the vocal folds cause dysphonia by limiting vocal fold closure and disrupting the mucosal wave. The size, site, number and type of lesion(s) will influence the severity of dysphonia and perceptual characteristics of the vocal quality.

## Principles of clinical practice in the management of mass lesions

In 2001, a survey of all active members of the American Academy of Otolaryngology–Head and Neck Surgery was conducted to determine opinion and practice for their management of benign vocal fold lesions (Sulica and Behrman, 2003). Participants were asked to indicate their treatment practices for benign vocal fold lesions, covering a range of possibilities including voice therapy, and to rate their frequency of use of a specific treatment or technique using a Likert 5-point scale. The response rate for the survey was 18.2%, with only 16.5% stating that they treated voice disorders: 30% of respondents indicated that they would choose voice therapy as an initial treatment for polyps with 22% electing for initial voice therapy for cysts. When considering voice therapy as an option in addition to surgery, either pre or post-operatively, the responses were spread across the Likert scale evenly (i.e. from "always" to "never").

Many authors recommend voice therapy pre and/or post-operatively for mass lesions (Bastian, 1996; Gallivan and Eitnier, 2006; Gallivan *et al.*, 2008; Lai *et al.*, 2013) often with adjunctive medical therapies such as anti-reflux medication, steroids and antibiotics. Johns advocates a trial of appropriate voice therapy for almost all cases of vocal lesions arising from vocal misuse before considering surgery (Johns, 2003). The rationale for offering voice therapy is that modifying hyperfunctional laryngeal behaviours reduces the vocal fold trauma that may have caused or contributed to the development of the lesion(s) (Hochman and Zeitels, 2000). A study by Andrade and colleagues (1999) found that hard glottal attack as a phonatory feature was significantly greater in dysphonic patients compared with a matched control group. This was the case for both muscle tension dysphonia and benign vocal fold lesions including cysts and nodules.

## Evidence for the effectiveness of voice therapy with a variety of mass lesions

A small number of studies have reported on voice therapy effectiveness in a broad range of patients which have included those with both functional and mass lesions (Bassiouny, 1998; Murry and Rosen, 2000; Casper, 2001; Rattenbury *et al.*, 2004). These studies have not attempted to separate the data with respect to pathological presentation and hence do not provide specific evidence of the effectiveness of voice therapy with mass lesions.

Cohen and Garrett (2007) carried out a retrospective review over a three year period of 57 patients with vocal fold polyps ($n$=41) and cysts ($n$= 16) who had received a course of voice therapy. Differentiation was made between translucent, haemorrhagic and fibrotic cysts as diagnosed by videolaryngostroboscopy. Patients had a mean age of 36 years (range 15–72 years) with a 22.8: 77.2% male to female ratio. A voice therapy programme was carried out by speech pathologists and/or singing specialists. Each programme was individually tailored to the patient's needs and included techniques for vocal hygiene, breath support, laryngeal tension and pitch. Patients were required to have attended a minimum of two speaking/singing voice therapy sessions to be included in the review but no detail is given on the maximum or average number of sessions or their frequency. Improvement in voice quality was defined as the patient indicating that their voice was sufficiently improved to meet their daily needs at the last therapy session. Voice improvement was achieved in 49% of patients and regardless of diagnosis. Three polyps and one cyst resolved entirely. Translucent polyps appeared to respond more favourably to voice therapy than haemorrhagic or fibrotic polyps. Although these results are encouraging, the measures on which the outcomes are based are limited. The use of an established self-report questionnaire along with perceptual and acoustic measures would have provided a more thorough evaluation of the effectiveness of voice therapy.

Schindler *et al.*, (2013) carried out a prospective study to investigate the multidimensional assessment of vocal changes in benign vocal fold lesions after voice therapy. A total of 65 consecutive patients (12 males and 53 females) presenting with Reinke's oedema ($n$=23), vocal cysts ($n$=22) and vocal polyps ($n$=20) were listed for phonosurgery. Prior to the surgery each participant was given 10 sessions of voice therapy, twice weekly. No additional pharmacological treatment was given. A range of pre and post-therapy outcome measures was used: The Voice Handicap Index (Jacobson *et al.*, 1997)no instruments exist to quantify the psychosocial consequences of voice disorders. The aim of the present investigation was the development of a statistically robust Voice Handicap Index (VHI, Maximum Phonation Time (MPT); acoustic analysis; perceptual rating using GIRBAS – a modified version of GRBAS (Hirano, 1982) and videolaryngostroboscopy (VLS). For the latter two measures the judges were blinded as to whether the recording shown was pre- or post-therapy. The voice therapy programme included general advice on voice production, elimination of voice misuse and vocal hygiene coupled with an individually tailored programme to reduce hyperkinetic laryngeal behaviours and encourage efficient vocal fold vibration. Post-therapy VLS demonstrated that there had been improvement in the appearance of 11 lesions (two Reinke's oedema; nine polyps) although none of the lesions had completely resolved. Improvement was judged as reduction by 50% or more in the size of the lesion. Of the other outcome measures, there was no reported difference in MPT, but significant differences were observed on the perceptual, acoustic and self-assessment ratings. Despite no lesions having completely resolved, only 40 of the 65 patients chose to proceed to phonosurgery (15 Reinke's oedema, 14 cysts and 11 polyps) while the other 25 were satisfied with their voice quality.

Tang and Thibeault (2016) investigated the timing of voice therapy intervention for patients (*n*= 29) who had surgery for a removal of a benign vocal fold lesion (including polyps, cysts and nodules). This was a retrospective review of information collected from a prospective outcomes database in a clinical setting. The review split cases into three categories as shown in Table 1.

Table 1: Voice Therapy Groups (Tang and Thibeault, 2016)

| Group | n | Benign vocal fold lesions |
| --- | --- | --- |
| Pre-operative (1 session of counselling plus post-op voice therapy) | 12 (M:6; F:6) | Polyp 8; Cyst 2 |
| Pre and post-operative voice therapy | 11 (M:3; F:8) | Polyp 4; Cyst 4; Nodules 2; Combination 2 |
| Post-operative voice therapy only | 8 (M:3; F:5) | Polyp 5; Cyst 1; Nodules 1: Combination 2 |

Pre-operative counselling consisted of advice on general vocal hygiene, immediate post-operative voice care and expectations of surgery. The voice therapy procedure is not specified other than as "direct voicing strategies". Outcome measures included the VHI self-report questionnaire and acoustic measures including jitter %, Dysphonia Severity Index scores (Hakkesteegt *et al.*, 2010) and noise to harmonics ratio (NHR). All post-operative measures were taken "within 4 months after the surgery" but it is unclear whether voice therapy had been completed at this point. There was no significant difference in any of the acoustic measures taken for any of the therapy groups. Inherent variability in acoustic measurements and small subject numbers means that it is not possible to draw any real conclusions with regard to the effectiveness of voice therapy. No auditory perceptual rating of voice quality was conducted. All three groups showed reduced average VHI scores but this only reached statistical significance for the two groups which had received pre-operative therapy intervention. These statistical differences were not related to the number of voice therapy sessions, only to whether therapy had occurred on one or more occasions *before* surgery.

## Evidence for the effectiveness of voice therapy for treating vocal polyps

Klein *et al.*, (2009) retrospectively reviewed the cases of 29 subjects diagnosed with true vocal fold haemorrhagic polyps. Of these, 13 patients had proceeded to immediate surgery while the other nine chose voice therapy and/or observation. All of the subjects choosing conservative treatment had "resolution" of their polyps over an average of 4.4 months (range 0.5–10 months). Conservative treatment included non-specified (in terms of either content or dosage) voice therapy and anti-reflux management via proton pump inhibitors and diet advice where appropriate. It is therefore difficult to draw any conclusions about the specific contribution of voice therapy.

Cho *et al.*, (2011) employed a retrospective review of hospital records to analyse the factors influencing voice quality and therapeutic approaches in patients with unilateral polyps. All patients ($n$= 202) diagnosed with a vocal fold polyp were offered voice therapy as a first line treatment. A total of 44 patients had declined therapy and undergone phonosurgery. The remaining 158 sets of records for patients who had attended for voice therapy were therefore reviewed. The aim of the voice therapy was to use strategies to reduce underlying vibratory trauma and maximise vocal efficiency. Techniques used included vocal hygiene, reduction of vocal abuse, breathing exercises and the Accent Method. Details of the voice therapy carried out in this study are limited with the number of sessions offered dependent on the severity of the voice disorder and patient compliance. Videolaryngostroboscopy was used to determine the size, location, position, colour and shape of the polyp before and after therapy. Other factors taken into account were vocal fold colour, reactive lesions on the contralateral fold, muscle tension dysphonia and laryngopharyngeal reflux.

Outcome measures also included perceptual assessment of voice quality (GRBAS), a self-report questionnaire (VHI) and acoustic measures (jitter, shimmer, noise-to-harmonic ratio). Videostroboscopy identified 104 patients in whome the polyp had reduced by at least 50% of its original size or completely resolved. The remaining 54 patients did not improve with therapy and required phonosurgical removal of the lesion. The study also evaluated which clinico-morphological factors affected the outcome of voice therapy. The size of the polyp and colour of the vocal fold were both statistically significant factors in the outcome of voice therapy. Patients with smaller polyps and whitish vocal folds had better outcomes than those with larger or reddish coloured vocal folds.

Nagakawa *et al.*, (2012) retrospectively reviewed the medical records of patients diagnosed with vocal fold polyps over a seven year period. Of 644 patients, 132 had received conservative treatment without surgical intervention. Conservative treatment was defined as voice therapy and/or medication. Voice therapy protocols were determined according to patient need and included counselling, vocal hygiene and breath support. Medication included steroid administration and/or steroid inhalation therapy. A large majority (71%) of these cases received medication therapy only. Only 29% of patients ($n= 38$) received voice therapy either in combination with medication ($n= 24$) or without medication ($n= 14$). Half (50%) of patients that received voice therapy with medication had complete resolution or shrinkage of the lesion whereas 43% of patients who had voice therapy with no medication had a similar outcome. The sole outcome measure used in this review was "size of lesion" as judged by the examining surgeon. No measures of vocal quality or patient reported outcomes were used. From the very small number who received voice therapy as part of the "conservative treatment" (29%) it is impossible to draw any definitive conclusions from this study as to the effectiveness of voice therapy with vocal fold polyps.

Lin *et al.*, (2014) report on a prospective study to assess the effect of voice rehabilitation in 60 patients who had undergone $CO_2$ laser surgery for unilateral vocal fold polyps. Subjects were randomly allocated to a voice training group or a control group. There were 33 male and 27 female study participants with an average age of 44.5 years (range 30–68 years). The method of randomisation is not described but each group had the same cultural background, degree of severity of dysphonia and course of disease. All patients had followed a post-operative voice rest programme, had taken advice on good vocal care and received a course of antibiotics and corticosteroids. The 30 participants in the training group then received a highly structured four week vocal rehabilitation programme including education on voice production as well as specific therapy techniques comprising relaxation, breath support, release of laryngopharyngeal constriction, chewing and phonation exercises. The programme delivered was exactly the same for each participant. Individual therapy sessions took place weekly with participants encouraged to practice between sessions. Further telephone support was provided as required.

A comprehensive range of pre and post-treatment outcome measures included GRBAS perceptual ratings of voice quality, Voice Handicap Index, aerodynamic measures (Maximum Phonation Time) and a range of acoustic measures (jitter, shimmer, pitch perturbation quotient, amplitude perturbation quotient and noise to harmonic ratio). Results showed that three months post-surgery all the outcome parameters for the vocal rehabilitation group were better than those in the control group and the difference was statistically significant ($p < 0.05$). This robust randomised controlled study with a clearly defined voice therapy programme and a range of outcome measures provides convincing evidence of voice therapy effectiveness for post-surgery intervention for patients with unilateral vocal fold polyps.

Petrovic-Lazic *et al.*, (2015) reported on a case series of 41 female patients (18–61 years; mean 47 years) with unilateral vocal fold polyps who were treated with both surgery and voice therapy. Perceptual and acoustic assessment of voice quality was performed pre-operatively and post-therapy. Acoustic data were also compared with age and sex matched normative data obtained concurrently at the same facility. The perceptual characteristics of the voice used a shortened version of the GRBAS scale (GRB only) and were rated by two speech-language pathologists and one laryngologist. It is unclear whether the GRB scores were averaged or whether a consensus was reached between raters. The acoustic measures consisted of fundamental frequency ($F_0$), fundamental frequency variation ($F_0v$), jitter, pitch perturbation quotient (PPQ), shimmer, amplitude perturbation quotient (APQ), noise to harmonic ratio (NHR) and voice turbulence index (VTI). Pre-operative acoustic assessment showed statistically significantly higher scores on all parameters for the polyp group than the control group. There was also significant positive correlation between the acoustic and perceptual voice parameters. Following phonosurgery, the acoustic measures showed a statistically significant improvement ($p < 0.01$) on all parameters except APQ and PPQ which only reached significance at $p > 0.05$. Perceptual measures after surgery are not reported. Participants then attended a therapy programme which included good vocal hygiene, reduction of vocal abuse and direct techniques to alter pitch, loudness and breath support as well as relaxation and stress reduction strategies. All participants had also received two sessions of voice therapy education prior to surgery. Each participant attended for therapy three times weekly for four weeks, beginning 10 days after surgery.

The authors report that following the course of voice therapy all perceptual voice measures (grade, breathiness and roughness) showed a statistically significant improvement. In addition they report significant improvement on the acoustic measures. It is unclear whether this is a further improvement from the findings post-surgery. The authors conclude that an improvement in voice quality is likely when carrying out a combination of phonosurgery and voice therapy for patients with vocal fold polyps. The lack of clarity regarding the exact timings of the assessments means that it is not possible to determine the relative benefit of the two components of intervention: surgery and voice therapy.

Zhuge et al., (2016) evaluated the changes in voice quality in patients with early vocal fold polyps before and after voice therapy. Inclusion criteria were specific: dysphonia lasting no more than six months with the presence of a unilateral or bilateral vocal fold polyp(s) at the anterior third with a diameter of no more than a quarter of the vocal fold. From a total of 88 eligible patients, 66 patients (M: 18; F: 48) completed the course of voice therapy. Each participant received three months of voice therapy, a 60–90 minute session every two to three weeks. The specific therapy programme included relaxation, breathing, vocal function exercises, resonance improvement, carryover techniques, prevention of misuse and vocal education. Following voice therapy, the polyp(s) had completely disappeared in 20 cases (30.3%) and had decreased in size in a further 35 (53%). They remained unchanged in the other 11 (11.6%). There was a statistically significant difference in the Voice Handicap Index (VHI) and Dysphonia Severity Index (DSI) before and after treatment.

## Effectiveness of voice therapy in treating vocal pseudocysts

Estes and Sulica (2014) carried out a retrospective cohort study in order to describe treatment results and identify predictors of the need for surgical intervention in patients with a pseudocyst of the vocal fold. They identified 46 patients (M: 5; F: 41) from a clinical database who had attended a course of voice therapy. None had undergone surgical intervention prior to the voice therapy. Patients had a mean age of 28.5 years with a range of 18 to 67 years. Therapy included vocal hygiene, education, reduction of maladaptive laryngeal tension, breathing techniques and healthy voice production. Patients attended between two and twelve weekly sessions with a mean of eight. On completion of voice therapy 29 (63%) of patients were "able to use their voice for their daily needs" and did not require surgery. Although the VHI-10 was used as an outcome measure it was not completed in all cases and no acoustic or perceptual measures were reported.

This is the only study where voice therapy has been evaluated as a sole treatment for vocal fold pseudocysts (where the diagnostic category is considered as a distinct mass lesion).

## Effectiveness of voice therapy with granuloma

Bloch *et al.*, performed an early study into the effect of voice therapy on contact granulomas of the vocal fold. This prospective study of 17 patients (age range 30–74) included nine who had received previous single or multiple surgeries and eight who had not undergone previous surgery. All participants had occupations requiring a heavy vocal load. Voice therapy was given weekly or less frequently with a total session ranging from 2 to 24 weeks. Voice therapy content was devised according to individual need but aimed to change the pattern of vocal fold vibration as well as taking into account psychological aspects of the voice disorder. Reduction of vocal abuse, breathing, relaxation and reduction in vocal tract tension were all employed as therapy techniques. Results were judged by the treating laryngologist and speech therapist based on laryngoscopic and auditory findings. Nine patients had complete elimination of the contact granuloma with a further four having a reduction in lesion size. Four patients were judged to have normal voices at the end of treatment while some improvement was noted in a further seven; six patients showed no change.

Ylilato and Hammarberg (2000) evaluated the laryngosocopic findings and voice characteristics of contact granuloma patients before and after voice therapy and at a nine year follow-up. This was a retrospective case series review of 19 male patients selected from 110 patients diagnosed with contact granuloma over a 17-year period. This is a convenience sample based on the availability of a pre-treatment, post-treatment and follow-up audio recording. Voice therapy was well described and included vocal hygiene, relaxation, posture and breath support work, reduction of vocal hyperfunction using the Accent Method, adjustment of speaking fundamental frequency and increasing pitch range. The mean number of voice therapy sessions was 26 with a range from 10 to 56. A range of vocal qualities was rated on a specifically designed visual analogue scale. Inter-rater reliability (five SLPs) was found to be satisfactory on all measures except diplophonia. The recordings were digitised and the acoustic parameters of $F_0$ and waveform perturbation were analysed. Following therapy, laryngeal examination indicated that 10 (52.6%) of the patients showed "healing" of the granuloma while the other nine showed no change. There was no significant change in either the perceptual ratings or acoustic measures post therapy.

Leonard and Kendall (2005) performed a retrospective review of 16 patients (M: 11; F: 5) presenting with unilateral and bilateral vocal process granuloma(s) who were offered a specific voice therapy treatment approach. All patients had previously received treatment for laryngopharyngeal or extra-oesophageal reflux for between six months and four years. Voice therapy included advice on voice production, vocal effort and anti-reflux lifestyle precautions and reflux medications. Patients were then offered voice therapy using a "phonoscopic" approach, by which the larynx is observed endoscopically by the patient whilst therapy techniques are carried out, allowing both visual and auditory feedback. The aim was to modify the vocal fold contact pattern leaving a small gap between the vocal processes. Therapy dosage ranged from five to eight sessions (mean = five) over a two to eight month period. Following therapy, a re-evaluation of the lesion(s) was performed by the laryngologist. Patients who were able to achieve the voice therapy technique goals experienced resolution or reduction in size of the granuloma(s). Phonatory function tests including measurements of maximum phonation time and airflow rates were also carried out pre- and post-therapy, but the findings are not reported on in detail.

The evidence of the effectiveness of voice therapy for treating granulomas is very limited due to the small number of studies, their level of study design and small participant numbers. No studies have demonstrated significant changes in either perceptual or acoustic measures. Evaluating the contribution of the voice therapy to improvement is often confounded by patients taking reflux medications at the same time.

A summary of all of the studies described above is presented in the Table below:

Table 2: Studies of Voice Treatment for Vocal Fold Mass Lesions

| First author | Type of study | Type of lesion | n | Type of treatment (inc duration and intensity) | Outcome Measures | Summary of Findings |
|---|---|---|---|---|---|---|
| Bloch et al., 1981 | Prospective cohort study | Contact granuloma | 17 | -Post-surgery voice therapy -Voice therapy programme described -Dosage: range from 2 to 24 sessions | Laryngoscopy Auditory rating of normality | 76% showed elimination or reduced lesion 4 voice returned to normal, 7 showed some improvement, 6 showed no change. No statistical analysis |
| Ylilato and Hammarberg, 2000 | Retrospective case series | Contact granuloma | 19 | -Voice therapy programme described -Dosage : range from 10 to 56 (mean = 26) | Auditory rating scale inter-rater reliability) $F_0$ Jitter Shimmer | No significant changes in any measures pre vs post therapy |
| Leonard and Kendall, 2005 | Retrospective review | Contact granuloma | 16 | "Phonoscopic" therapy Dosage: 5–8 sessions (mean 5) over a 2–8 month period | Laryngoscopy MPT Airflow rates | Reduced size of lesion No other measures reported No statistical analysis |
| Cohen and Garrett, 2007 | Retrospective review | Polyps and cysts | 57 | -Individually tailored programme - No details of dosage | Patient self-rating of improvement | 49% improved No statistical analysis |
| Klein et al., 2009 | Retrospective review | Haemorrhagic vocal fold polyps | 29 | No details of content of dosage | Laryngostroboscopy | "Resolution" of polyps over an average of 4.4 months |

| First author | Type of study | Type of lesion | n | Type of treatment (inc duration and intensity) | Outcome Measures | Summary of Findings |
|---|---|---|---|---|---|---|
| Cho et al., 2011 | Retrospective review | Unilateral vocal fold polyps | 158 | -Description of techniques<br>-Dosage dependent on severity of presentation | Laryngostroboscopy<br>GRBAS<br>VHI<br>Jitter, shimmer and NHR | -66% showed reduced lesion size or resolved<br>Grade is significantly correlated with jitter/shimmer<br>Multivariate linear regression analysis shows size of polyp to be the only factor to affect vocal quality |
| Nakagawa et al., 2012 | Retrospective review | Vocal fold polyps | 38 | -Undefined voice therapy programme<br>-No details of dosage | Laryngostroboscopy (size of lesion) | 43, 50% of patients who received voice therapy showed improvement<br>No statistical analysis |
| Schindler et al., 2013 | Prospective cohort study | Reinke's oedema, polyps and cysts | 65 | -Well described treatment programme<br>-10 sessions (twice a week) | VHI<br>MPT<br>GIRBAS<br>Acoustic analysis<br>Laryngostroboscopy (VLS) | -Significant difference in acoustic analysis, GIRBAS and VHI<br>-No significant difference in MPT and VLS. |
| Lin et al., 2014 | Prospective pseudo-randomised trial (post-surgery) | Vocal fold polyps | 60 | -No treatment control group<br>-Highly structured voice therapy protocol<br>-Dosage: 1 x 4 weeks | VHI<br>GRBAS<br>Jitter<br>Shimmer<br>PPQ<br>APQ<br>NHR<br>MPT | Statistically significant differences between voice therapy intervention group and control group. |

| First author | Type of study | Type of lesion | n | Type of treatment (inc duration and intensity) | Outcome Measures | Summary of Findings |
|---|---|---|---|---|---|---|
| Estes and Sulica, 2014 | Retrospective cohort study | Pseudocyst | 46 | | | |
| Petrovic-Lazic et al., 2015 | Case series | Vocal fold polyps | 41 | -Surgery and voice therapy. -Voice therapy programme described in detail -Dosage: 3 x 4 weeks | GRB (only) F0 Jitter PPQ Shimmer APQ NHR VTI | Statistically significant improvement in all a parameters ($p > 0.05$) |
| Tang and Thibeault, 2016 | Retrospective review | Polyps, cysts and nodules | 29 | -Indirect therapy described -Content of direct therapy not specified --No details of dosage | VHI Jitter Shimmer Dysphonia Severity index NHR | -No significant difference in any acoustic measures - Significant difference in VHI for patients who received pre-operative therapy |
| Zhuge et al., 2016 | Prospective cohort study | "Early" unilateral and bilateral vocal fold polyps | 66 | -No surgery -Specific voice therapy programme -Dosage: 60–90 minute session every 2–3 weeks for 3 months | VHI DSI | Statistically significant ($p = >0.05$) difference pre vs post-treatment in VHI and DSI |

Abbreviations: $F_0$ = Fundamental Frequency, PPQ= Pitch Perturbation Quotient, APQ = Amplitude Perturbation Quotient, NHR = Noise to Harmonic Ratio, VTI = Voice Turbulence Index, DSI = Dyshonia Severity Index, VHI = Voice Handicap Index, MPT= Maximum Phonation Time.

## Summary

The main problem in evaluating the efficacy of voice therapy for the management of mass lesions is that behavioral intervention is often used as part of a combination of treatments. This combination usually includes surgical intervention and/or reflux medication. This reflects the lack of understanding of the aetiology of many vocal fold mass lesions (and hence a lack of clarity about how to treat them) or, at least, an acknowledgement that the causation may be multi-factorial. It is therefore appropriate that most of the studies have been retrospective reviews or case series (Level IV evidence), often with small numbers. There is only a small number of more recently emerging studies providing Level III evidence (Schindler *et al.*, 2013; Lin *et al.*, 2014; Zhuge *et al.*, 2016). This corresponds to Robey's Phase 1 (see Chapter 2) which is described as follows (Robey, 2004):

- Aiming to detect the presence of a therapeutic effect by using single case studies, small-group studies and retrospective studies
- Research that explores and specifies the therapeutic effect as the main dependent variable
- Detection of an effect that would provide justification of further investigation.

Studies which have evaluated a combination of interventions and that also have small patient numbers and limited methodology are unable to isolate the effectiveness of the voice therapy intervention itself.

Furthermore the outcome measures used in many of these studies were commonly unsophisticated and subject to significant bias. The visual (laryngoscopic) and auditory (voice quality) judgements were poorly defined, rarely used standard tools or procedures, and were commonly judged by clinicians involved in the patients treatment (with no inter-or intra-judge reliability reporting). This is especially the case in the retrospective reviews. However, a small number of studies has clearly defined parameters for making these judgements and employed multiple raters using either inter-rater reliability or consensus ratings. Some have used judges blinded to whether they are rating pre or post treatment. Five studies used multidimensional outcome measures. A further common problem was the lack of clarity regarding the timing of the outcome measurements making it impossible to determine the relative value of different components of a sequential programme of therapy. For example, as studies involving consecutive surgery and therapy rarely reported the findings between the two interventions, it was difficult to differentiate the relative effect of each intervention.

However, it is important to observe that there is some emerging Level III evidence that voice therapy can be effective in the management of mass lesions of the vocal folds often in combination with other forms of management such as surgery or medication. The strongest evidence points to voice therapy intervention with polyps either following surgery (Lin *et al.*, 2014) or for early polyps as the primary treatment (Zhuge *et al.*, 2016). Future prospective studies would enable an evaluation of the effectiveness of voice therapy with mass lesions using multidimensional outcome measures immediately before and after therapy, with longer term follow-up.

# References

Andrade DF, Heuer R, Hockstein NE, *et al.* (1999) The frequency of hard glottal attacks in patients with muscle tension dysphonia, unilateral benign masses and bilateral benign masses. *Journal of Voice* 14(2): 240–246.

Arens C, Glanz H and Kleinsasser, O (1997) Clinical and morphological aspects of laryngeal cysts. *European Archives of Oto-Rhino-Laryngology* 254: 430–436.

Bassiouny S (1998) Efficacy of the Accent Method of Voice Therapy. *Folia Phoniatrica et Logopaedica* 50: 146–164.

Bastian RW (1996) Vocal fold microsurgery in singers. *Journal of Voice* 10(4): 389–404.

Bloch C, Gould WJ, Hirano M (1981). Effect of voice therapy on contact granuloma of the vocal fold. *Annals of Otology, Rhinology and Laryngology* 90(1): 48–52.

Carroll TL, Gartner-Schmidt J, Statham MM and Rosen CA (2010) Vocal process granuloma and glottal insufficiency: an overlooked etiology? *The Laryngoscope* 120(1): 114–120.

Casper J (2001) Treatment outcomes in occupational voice disorders. In: P. Dejonckere (Ed.) *Occupational Voice: Care and Cure.* The Hague: Kugler Publications, pp 187–199.

Cho KJ, Nam IC, Hwang YS *et al.* (2011) Analysis of factors influencing voice quality and therapeutic approaches in vocal polyp patients. *European Archives of Oto-Rhino-Laryngology* 268(9): 1321–1327.

Cohen SM and Garrett CG (2007) Utility of voice therapy in the management of vocal fold polyps and cysts. *Otolaryngology - Head and Neck Surgery* (136): 742–746.

Colton RH, Woo P, Brewer DW *et al.* (1995) Stroboscopic signs associated with benign lesions of the vocal folds. *Journal of Voice* 9(3): 312–325.

Cornut G, Bouchayer M and Parent F (1986) Value of videostroboscopy in indicating phonosurgery. *Acta Otorhinolaryngologica Belgica* 40: 436–442.

Estes C and Sulica L (2014) Vocal fold pseudocyst: results of 46 cases undergoing a uniform treatment algorithm. *The Laryngoscope* 124(5): 1180–1186.

Gallivan G, Gallivan H and Eitnier C (2008). Dual intracordal unilateral vocal fold cysts: a perplexing diagnostic and therapeutic challenge. *Journal of Voice* 22(1): 119–124.

Gallivan GJ and Eitnier CM (2006) Vocal fold polyp in a professional brass/wind instrumentalist and singer. *Journal of Voice* 20(1): 157–164.

Hakkesteegt MM, Brocaar MP and Wieringa MH (2010) The applicability of the Dysphonia Severity Index and the Voice Handicap Index in evaluating effects of voice therapy and phonosurgery. *Journal of Voice* 24: 199–205.

Hirano M (1982) *Clinical Examination of Voice* London: Springer-Verlag.

Hochman I and Zeitels S (2000) Phonomicrosurgical management of vocal fold polyps: the subepithelial microflap resection technique. *Journal of Voice* 14(1): 112–118.

Jacobson BH, Johnson A and Grywalski C (1997) The Voice Handicap Index (VHI): development and validation. *American Journal of Speech-Language Pathology* 6: 66–69.

Johns MM (2003) Update on the etiology, diagnosis and treatment of vocal fold nodules, polyps and cysts. *Current Opinion in Otolaryngology & Head and Neck Surgery* 11: 456–461.

Klein A, Lehmann M, Hapner ER and Johns MM III *et al.* (2009). Spontaneous resolution of hemorrhagic polyps of the true vocal fold. *Journal of Voice* 23(1): 132–135.

Koufman JA, Belafsky PC and Forest W (2001). Unilateral or localized Reinke's Edema (pseudocyst) as a manifestation of vocal fold paresis: the paresis nodule. *The Laryngoscope* 111(4 Pt 1): 576–580.

Lai Y-T Petty BE, Huang W, Dailey SH (2013). Bilateral vocal fold chondromas. *Journal of Voice* 27(2): 255–257.

Leonard R and Kendall K (2005) Effects of voice therapy on vocal process granuloma: a phonoscopic approach. *American Journal of Otolaryngology* 26(2): 101–107.

Lin L, Sun N, Yang Q *et al.* (2014) Effect of voice training in the voice rehabilitation of patients with vocal cord polyps after surgery. *Experimental and Therapeutic Medicine* 7(4): 877–880.

Martins RH, Defaveri J, Domingues MA and de Albuquerque e Silva R. (2011a) Vocal polyps: clinical, morphological, and immunohistochemical aspects. *Journal of Voice* 25(1): 98–106.

Martins RHG, Santana MF and Tavares ELM (2011b) Vocal cysts: clinical, endoscopic, and surgical aspects. *Journal of Voice* 25(1): 107–110.

Martins RHG, Dias NH, Santos DC *et al.* (2009). Clinical, histological and electron microscopic aspects of vocal fold granulomas. *Brazilian Journal of Otorhinolaryngology* 75(1): 116–122.

Murry T and Rosen C (2000) Outcome measurements and quality of life in voice disorders. *Otolaryngologic Clinics of North America* 33: 905–916.

Nakagawa H, Miyamoto M, Kusuyama T *et al.*, 2012. Resolution of vocal fold polyps with conservative treatment. *Journal of voice*, 26(3), pp.e107–10.

Petrovic-Lazic M, Jovanovic N, Kulic M *et al.* (2015). Acoustic and perceptual characteristics of the voice in patients with vocal polyps after surgery and voice therapy. *Journal of Voice* **29**(2): 241–246.

Rattenbury HJ, Carding PN and Finn P (2004) Evaluating the effectiveness and efficiency of voice therapy using transnasal flexible laryngoscopy: a randomized controlled trial. *Journal of Voice* **18**(4): 522–533.

Robey RR (2004) A five-phase model for clinical outcome research. *Journal of Communication Disorders* **37**: 401–411

Rosen, C., Gartner-Schmidt, J. and Hathaway, B., 2012. A nomenclature paradigm for benign midmembranous vocal fold lesions. *The Laryngoscope*, 122, pp.1335–1341.

Schindler A, Mozzanica F, Maruzzi P *et al.* (2013) Multidimensional assessment of vocal changes in benign vocal fold lesions after voice therapy. *Auris Nasus Larynx* **40**: 291–297.

Sulica L and Behrman A (2003) Management of benign vocal fold lesions: A survey of current opinion and practice. *Annals of Otology, Rhinology and Laryngology* **112**(10): 827–833.

Tan M and Pitman MJ (2011) A case of bilateral vocal fold mucosal bridges, bilateral trans-vocal fold type III sulci vocales, and an intracordal polyp. *Journal of Voice* **25**(4): 484–486.

Tang SS and Thibeault SL (2016) Timing of voice therapy: a primary investigation of voice outcomes for surgical benign vocal fold lesion patients. *Journal of Voice* (In Press).

Ylitalo R and Hammarberg B (2000) Voice characteristics, effects of voice therapy, and long-term follow-up of contact granuloma patients. *Journal of Voice* **14**(4): 557–566.

Zhuge P, You H, Wang H *et al* (2016) An analysis of the effects of voice therapy on patients with early vocal fold polyps. *Journal of Voice* (In press).

# 6

# The effectiveness of voice therapy for patients with unilateral vocal fold paralysis

## Chloe Walton and Paul Carding

## Introduction

Unilateral vocal fold paralysis (UVFP) arises from a loss of innervation to one of the branches in the recurrent laryngeal nerve. The recurrent laryngeal nerve (RLN) innervates all of the intrinsic muscles of the larynx with the exception of the cricothyroid muscle. Disruption to the RLN results in immobility to one of the vocal folds, resulting in glottal incompetence due to poor vocal fold adduction (Woodson, 2008; Zealear and Billante, 2004). This typically results in dysphonia and occasionally dysphagia. Given its recurrent nature and length, the left branch of the RLN is susceptible to injury; this may be due to a wide range of aetiology including neoplasms, traumatic injury, neurological diseases, iatrogenic or idiopathic causes (Havas *et al.*, 1999). The severity of these injuries varies depending on aetiology and can be classified into three types: neuropraxia (temporary block of nerve impulses); axonotmesis (a disruption or cutting of the axon leading to paralysis in the motor and sensory systems); or neurotmesis (severe nerve damage where the entire nerve fibre is cut or damaged, resulting in a complete loss of motor, sensory and automatic function). The more severe the injury, the more likely that recovery will only be partial and limited (Sittel *et al.*, 2001).

People with UVFP typically experience perceptually hoarse, weak voices with associated vocal fatigue and potentially breathing and swallowing difficulties (Paniello et al., 2011; Seyed Toutounchi et al., 2014). UVFP can have a significant impact on a patient's quality of life in a number of functional, physiological and emotional domains (D'Alatri et al., 2008). This can lead to further problems associated with stress and depression (Spector et al., 2001).

## Options of intervention for UVFP

The optimal aim of treatment for UVFP is to restore functional voicing and improve glottic insufficiency (Zealear and Billante, 2004). Currently, management of UVFP is either:

(1) surgical intervention and/or
(2) speech therapy (voice) exercises or
(3) wait for potential spontaneous recovery.

Typically, the management of UVFP is influenced by the following factors: presence of aspiration, nerve injury, nasoendoscopic findings, vocal demands, comorbidities, EMG findings and participant concerns (Rickert et al., 2012; Sulica, 2008). Depending on the above factors, participants may receive one or a combination of management options for their UVFP.

Voice therapy aims to improve e perceptual vocal quality and vocal endurance through the implementation of direct and indirect treatment techniques. Direct treatment targets specific voicing factors including: respiration, phonation and resonance. Indirect treatment targets vocal hygiene, environmental and personal factors which can influence voice quality and performance (D'Alatri et al., 2008; Miller, 2004).

This chapter reports on the evidence base for speech therapy intervention for UVFP and presents a critical evaluation of the literature. More specifically, the evaluation of the literature will be conducted through the rating of studies according to the NRMRC –levels of evidence (Intervention) (1999), the phase of research development Robey (2004) and a detailed critical appraisal.

## Identifying the evidence base of speech therapy effectiveness for treating UVFP

We searched seven electronic databases including: PubMed, Embase, CINHAL, Web of Science, Scopus, CENTRAL and Medline. The search was limited to human studies but no language or time restrictions were applied. Articles in the search were assessed based on the following inclusion criteria: adult participants between the ages of 18 and 70; confirmed diagnosis of UVFP; presence of dysphonia; intervention provided by a speech pathologist; studies with pre-/post-outcome data. Editorials and review articles (i.e., no intervention data) were excluded. The reference lists of the selected papers were also searched for additional literature. Inclusion and exclusion criteria for further critical analysis of the studies are listed in Table 1.

Table 1: Studies of Voice Treatment for Unilateral Vocal Fold Paralysis

| Authors | Number of Participants | Level of Evidence (NHMRC, 1999) | Treatment and Duration/Intensity | Outcome Measures | Findings |
|---|---|---|---|---|---|
| **Phase 1 studies (Robey, 2004)** | | | | | |
| Kelchner et al, 1999 | 117 | Retrospective case series – pre-/post-test Level IV | Treatment not described 1–13 sessions | Videolaryngoscope Unpublished 7 point perceptual rating scale | Voice therapy alone – no improvement Voice therapy + Medialisation = statistically significant change ($p < 0.05$) |
| Khidr, 2003 | 3 | Prospective case series – pre-/post-test Level IV | Smith Accent method Two 60 min sessions/week for 8 weeks | Videostrobe, MPT, GRBAS, VHI | All improved (no statistics reported) |
| D'Altri et al., 2008 | 30 | Prospective case series – pre-/post-test Level IV | Individualised programme Two 30 min sessions/week, 8 to 35 sessions | Videostrobe, MPT, Jitter, Shimmer, NHR, GRBAS $F_0$ | All showed statistically significant improvement ($p < 0.05$) apart from $F_0$ |
| Schindler et al., 2008 | 40 | Retrospective case series – pre-/post-test Level IV | Individualised programme Two sessions/week for 6 to 20 sessions | Videolaryngoscope MPT, GRIBAS, Shimmer, VHI, Jitter, NHR, Spectrographic $F_0$ | All showed statistically significant improvement ($p < 0.05$) apart from $F_0$ |
| Mattioli et al., 2011 | 74 | Prospective case series – pre-/post-test Level IV | 2 phased approach Two sessions/week for 14–20 sessions | Videostrobe MPT, $F_0$, Shimmer, Jitter, NHR | All showed statistically significant improvement ($p < 0.05$) (No videostrobe statistics) |

| Authors | Number of Participants | Level of Evidence (NHMRC, 1999) | Treatment and Duration/Intensity | Outcome Measures | Findings |
|---|---|---|---|---|---|
| Garcia Perez et al., 2014 | 10 | Prospective case series – pre-/post-test Level IV | Electrical stimulation with sustained phonation 1 x 30 min session for 10 sessions | Videostrobe MPT, Jitter, Shimmer, NHR, NNE $F_0$ | All showed statistically significant improvement ($p$ <0.05) (No videostrobe statistics) |
| Mattioli et al., 2015 | 171 | Retrospective case series – pre-/post-test Level IV | 2 phases: Forcible exercise with manipulations and manoeuvres Two sessions/week for 12–18 sessions | Videostrobe MPT, $F_0$, Jitter and NHR Shimmer | All showed statistically significant improvement ($p$ <0.05) (No videostrobe statistics) |
| Phase 2 studies (Robey, 2004) | | | | | |
| McFarlane et al., 1991 | 16 | Prospective concurrent control Level III -2 | Head turning Digital manipulation Half-swallow boom Range 3–24 hours of therapy | 1. Voice quality ratings (self-devised scale) | No change and no statistics reported |
| Cantarella et al., 2010 | 30 | Prospective quasi-experimental design III -2 | Individual therapy programme (not detailed) Range 10 to 40 sessions of therapy | 1. Voice quality ratings (self-devised scale) | Both treatment groups improved (no statistical analysis) |
| Colton et al., 2011 | 26 | Prospective quasi-experimental design III -2 | 4 to 6 sessions Details not specified | Unpublished dysphonia scale | Severity of dysphonia decreased in both groups ($p$ = <0.05) |

| Authors | Number of Participants | Level of Evidence (NHMRC, 1999) | Treatment and Duration/Intensity | Outcome Measures | Findings |
|---|---|---|---|---|---|
| El-Banna and Youseff, 2014 | 42 | Prospective quasi-experimental design III -2 | Pushing exercises Hard glottal attack Accent method No duration/intensity data given | Videostrobe GRBAS Dysphonia Severity Index | Early treatment group showed statistically significant improvement ($p = <0.05$) Late treatment group showed no statistically significant improvement |
| Busto-Cresspo et al., 2015 | 70 | Prospective quasi-experimental design III -2 | Pulmonary Function Voice source exercises Articulation 15 ×30 min sessions twice weekly | Videostrobe MPT Spectrographic VHI -10 Jitter Shimmer, NHR, $F_0$ | Statistically significant improvement ($p = <.05$) for Group 1 and Group 2 for some measures Group 1 improved more than Group 2 ($p = <0.05$) for some measures |

Assessment key: MPT – maximum phonation time, $F_0$ – fundamental frequency, Jitter – cycle-to-cycle variations of fundamental frequency (Hz) , Shimmer – cycle-to-cycle variations of amplitude (dB), NHR – Noise to harmonic ratio, vAm – variation's coefficient of amplitude, DUV – degree of unsounded voice, NNE – normalised noise energy, VHI – voice handicap index, VHI-10 – voice handicap index 10, VPSS – voice problem self-assessment scale, GRBAS – perceptual rating scale (Grade, roughness, breathiness, asthenia, strain), GRIBAS – perceptual rating scale (Grade, roughness, irregularity, breathiness, asthenia, strain), DSI – Dysphonia Severity Index.

## Study design

The 12 included studies represent a variety of study designs and the current levels of evidence according (NHMRC, 1999) for speech pathology management of UVFP. The highest level of evidence for speech pathology management of UVFP was identified as Level III-2 (El-Banna and Youssef, 2014). This study used two treatment groups and a no-treatment control group. The four remaining Level III studies were all classified as III-3 on the NHMRC hierarchy because they used comparative interventions but not controls (Busto-Crespo et al., 2015; Cantarella et al., 2010; Colton et al., 2011; McFarlane et al., 1991).

The remaining seven studies listed in the table above, all classified as Level IV (NHMRC, 1999), comprised all case series and reported pre- and post-outcome data (Kelchner et al., 1999; Khidr, 2003; D'Altri et al., 2008; Schindler et al., 2008; Mattioli et al., 2011; Garcia Perez et al., 2014; Mattioli et al., 2015).

## Participants

There was considerable heterogeneity in the studies with respect to participant characteristics. The five Level III studies reported on voice therapy outcomes for 184 participants with the total number of participants in each study varying from 16 to 70. Of the Level III participant data available there were 103 females and 71 males with an age range of 15 to 80 years. Two studies (Cantarella et al., 2010; McFarlane et al., 1991) included participants under 18 years of age; these studies were included in the review (despite the stated exclusion criteria) as there was no way of determining the number of participants in this age category. Interestingly, the diagnosis of UVFP was confirmed by stroboscopy in only three of the studies (Busto-Crespo et al., 2015; Cantarella et al., 2010; El-Banna and Youssef, 2014) and the diagnostic process was not described in the two studies (Colton et al., 2011; McFarlane et al., 1991). A total of four studies documented aetiological information (Busto-Crespo et al., 2015; Cantarella et al., 2010; Colton et al., 2011; El-Banna and Youssef, 2014) and a description of the side of paralysis (i.e., left vs right) was only reported for three studies (Cantarella et al., 2010; El-Banna and Youssef, 2014; McFarlane et al., 1991). The position of the UVFP (i.e., paramedian vs median) was documented in the two most recent studies (Busto-Crespo et al., 2015; El-Banna and Youssef, 2014) only. This lack of diagnostic information limits judgement of patient homogeneity in the studies and thus makes it difficult to determine whether these factors are important variables in treatment outcome.

The majority of Level IV studies were seen to have much higher participant numbers than the Level III studies, with a total of 494 participants and a range of 3 to 171 participants per study. Similar to the Level III studies there was a 34% male /66% female distribution and an age range from12 to 91 years. Two studies included participants younger than 18 years of age (Kelchner *et al.*, 1999; Khidr, 2003; Mattioli *et al.*, 2011; Schindler *et al.*, 2008) but were included in this review because it was not possible to determine how many participants in each study were younger thanthis. All seven Level IV studies reported aetiology of the paralysis and similar to the Level III studies, the most common aetiology of the UVFP was iatrogenic. Only two Level IV studies reported the side of the paralysis (Kelchner *et al.*, 1999; Khidr, 2003). Overall, participants included in the Level IV studies demonstrated characteristics similar to those in the Level III studies

## Voice therapy interventions

The published studies showed considerable variability in therapy content, timing of intervention and therapy duration.

### Therapy content

The therapy techniques used within the Levels III and IV studies varied greatly and involved a range of direct and indirect treatments. Only one study used a treatment protocol (Busto-Crespo *et al.*, 2015), despite being an established method of controlling this key study variable. In the study in question, therapy consisted of three treatment phases focusing on different subsystems of voicing: (1) positioning and respiration, (2) voicing through vocal exercises, humming, compression and cough attack and (3) voice projection, singing and biofeedback. The two Mattioli *et al.* studies (2011 and 2015) described two phases of treatment, one focused on vocal fold movement and the other on voice quality. These studies used a combination of voice therapy techniques including coughing with voicing, vocal function exercises and laryngeal manipulation and other manoeuvres to achieve glottal closure. The remaining Level III and IV studies used individualised treatment approaches with various combinations of direct therapy techniques focusing on respiratory, laryngeal and resonatory subsystems (Cantarella *et al.*, 2010; Colton *et al.*, 2011; D'Alatri *et al.*, 2008; McFarlane *et al.*, 1991; Schindler *et al.*, 2008). Treatment techniques included: half-swallow boom, Smith Accent Method, pushing exercises and glottal attack (Cantarella *et al.*, 2010; Colton *et al.*, 2011; El-Banna and Youssef, 2014; McFarlane *et al.*, 1991). There were two studies which made no reference to the therapy received by patients with UVFP (Colton *et al.*, 2011; Kelchner *et al.*, 1999). Theoretically the major value of Levels III and IV studies is to focus on clear and detailed intervention approaches which can be tested more formally in controlled designs (Robey, 2004). Therefore, we must conclude that there is no consensus and no homogeneity in the literature regarding therapy content, so further research is required focusing on specific therapy techniques to develop the understanding of optimal voice therapy management of UVFP.

## Therapy timing and duration

Several studies reported "early" commencement of speech therapy intervention (Kelchner *et al.*, 1999; Busto-Crespo *et al.*, 2015; Cantarella *et al.*, 2010; D'Alatri *et al.*, 2008; El-Banna and Youssef, 2014; Mattioli *et al.*, 2015; Schindler *et al.*, 2008). However, there was significant variation as to the definition of "early" commencement, varying from "within four weeks post diagnosis" (Kelchner *et al.*, 1999; Mattioli *et al.*, 2015) to "less than one year post onset" (Busto-Crespo *et al.*, 2015). Similarly, "late" commencement could vary from "more than 3 months" (Cantarella *et al.*, 2010) to "greater than 12 months post onset of UVFP" (Busto-Crespo *et al.*, 2015). Two studies did not examine or describe time post-onset when voice treatment was commenced (Colton *et al.*, 2011; McFarlane *et al.*, 1991).

Duration of treatment also differed between participants within each study and across studies. Two Level III studies addressed this variable, where intervention was specifically controlled to 15 sessions, 30 minutes twice weekly (Busto-Crespo *et al.*, 2015) and 10 sessions of electrical stimulation to target glottal insufficiency (Garcia Perez *et al.*, 2014) respectively. El-Banna and Youssef (2014) reported using the Smith Accent method for 16 sessions, 30 minutes twice weekly; however, they additionally reported some hard glottal attack and pushing exercises so total treatment duration is unclear. Over all of the Level III and IV studies, the range of total therapy sessions varied from one to 40 sessions. Only two studies reported home practice for participants (Cantarella *et al.*, 2010; Mattioli *et al.*, 2011). The majority of studies described a twice-weekly treatment regime (D'Alatri *et al.*, 2008; El-Banna and Youssef, 2014; Khidr, 2003; Mattioli *et al.*, 2015; Schindler *et al.*, 2008). Three studies made no reference to the intensity of treatment provided (Colton *et al.*, 2011; Kelchner *et al.*, 1999; McFarlane *et al.*, 1991).

## Effectiveness of treatment

Overall, the 12 studies suggest that voice therapy may be effective in improving voice quality and voice durability in patients with UVFP. Several studies also suggest that additional parameters, such as timing and frequency, may also contribute to the success of treatment. Furthermore, there is a trend suggesting that earlier intervention may be more effective for participants. However, the quality of this evidence is weak, with no study designs that incorporate prospective group analysis and that also include a controlled no treatment group. Also, details of diagnostic characteristics, treatment content and duration and levels of pre- and post-treatment outcome measures are very variable and commonly non-specific.

## Phase 1 efficacy studies

A number of Phase 1 case series studies reported perceptual, physiological and acoustic improvements post-voice therapy using a wide range of treatment techniques (Kelchner *et al.*, 1999; Khidr, 2003; D'Altri *et al.*, 2008; Schindler *et al.*, 2008; Mattioli *et al.*, 2011; Garcia Perez *et al.*, 2014; Mattioli *et al.*, 2015). In total, 494 cases were assessed, with several studies reporting on more than 100 cases (Kelchner *et al.*, 1999; Mattioli, 2015). A number of these studies provide multi-dimensional outcome data showing statistically significant change pre- and post-speech therapy intervention (D'Altri *et al.*, 2008; Schindler *et al.*, 2008; Mattioli *et al.*, 2011; Garcia Perez *et al.*, 2014; Mattioli *et al.*, 2015). Single case and case series studies can be very valuable for determining proof of concept and describing treatment in detail. This weight of case series material certainly appears to demonstrate that voice therapy can have a beneficial effect for patients with UVFP. However, details of therapy content remain elusive. Most of the studies illustrated individualised treatment approaches with various combinations of direct therapy techniques focusing on respiratory, laryngeal and resonatory subsystems. The specific details were often difficult to determine and would not be sufficient to allow replication. However, the two Mattioli *et al.* studies (2011 and 2015) did describe two phases of treatment, the first focused on vocal fold movement and the second on voice quality, which may be seen as a structure for future use.

## Phase 2 efficacy studies

A number of Phase 2 study designs (Robey, 2004) have investigated the efficacy of various forms of therapy using group comparisons (Busto-Crespo *et al.*, 2015; Cantarella *et al.*, 2010; Colton *et al.*, 2011; McFarlane *et al.*, 1991). Despite the significant weaknesses in these as highlighted above, two studies contain a number of positive features which could form the basis of future studies of speech therapy effectiveness for patients with UVFP (Busto-Crespo *et al.*, 2015; El-Banna and Youssef, 2014). El-Banna and Youssef (2014) provided a detailed prescriptive treatment protocol and employed a multi-dimensional assessment battery to demonstrate accurate comparisons of treatment outcomes. Furthermore, the authors reported on 42 participants with a defined age range and clear diagnostic homogeneity. Intensity and duration of treatment was also defined as 20-minute sessions, twice weekly over 8 weeks.

A recent study by Busto-Crespo *et al.*, (2015) also provides valuable data concerning treatment efficacy on 70 participants with UVFP. They report statistically significant pre- vs post-treatment change immediately after treatment and, for 32 participants, at one year follow-up. The use of a well-defined treatment protocol that contained a combination of direct and indirect techniques is a valuable contribution which may be utilised in future studies.

## Conclusions

This chapter aimed to analyse the current evidence for the speech pathology management for patients with UVFP. Overall, twelve studies were identified, with five studies being graded at Level III evidence (NHMRC 1999) and seven at Level IV. Despite the lack of homogeneity observed for recruitment, assessment and treatment, these studies do provide some evidence of treatment efficacy requiring further development. Some clarity of developed treatment protocols and intensity, timing and frequency are emerging (e.g., Busto-Crespo *et al.*, 2015). Longer term follow-up data (e.g., one year post-treatment) would be of great value but are acknowledged to be difficult to achieve with this population. There have been no studies that have attempted to determine the "value added" of voice therapy when it is applied following (or preceding) surgical intervention. Researchers may develop a stronger evidence base by building on preliminary studies. It is a refining process in evidence collection which results in the application of stronger design and consequently higher levels of evidence of treatment efficacy (Robey, 2004).

# References

Busto-Crespo O, Uzcanga-Lacabe M, Abad-Marco A *et al.* (2015) Longitudinal voice outcomes after voice therapy in unilateral vocal fold paralysis *Journal of Voice* doi: 10.1016/j.jvoice.2015.10.018

Cantarella G, Viglione S, Forti S, Pignataro L (2010) Voice therapy for laryngeal hemiplegia: the role of timing of initiation of therapy *Journal of Rehabilitation Medicine* 42(5): 442–446. doi: 10.2340/16501977–0540

Colton RH, Paseman A, Kelley RT *et al.* (2011) Spectral moment analysis of unilateral vocal fold paralysis *Journal of Voice* 25(3): 330–336. doi: 10.1016/j.jvoice.2010.03.006

D'Alatri L, Galla S, Rigante M *et al.* (2008) Role of early voice therapy in patients affected by unilateral vocal fold paralysis *Journal of Laryngology and Otology* 122(9): 936–941. doi: 10.1017/s0022215107000679

El-Banna M, Youssef G. (2014) Early voice therapy in patients with unilateral vocal fold paralysis *Folia Phoniatrica et Logopaedica* 66(6): 237–243.

Garcia Perez A, Hernandez Lopez X, Valadez Jimenez V *et al.* (2014) Synchronous electrical stimulation of laryngeal muscles: an alternative for enhancing recovery of unilateral recurrent laryngeal nerve paralysis *Journal of Voice* 28(4): e521–527. doi: 10.1016/j.jvoice.2014.01.004

Havas T, Lowinger D, Priestley J (1999) Unilateral vocal fold paralysis: causes, options and outcomes *The Australian and New Zealand Journal of Surgery* 69(7): 509–513.

Kelchner LN, Stemple JC, Gerdeman E *et al.* (1999) Etiology, pathophysiology, treatment choices and voice results for unilateral adductor vocal fold paralysis: a 3-year retrospective *Journal of Voice* 13(4): 592–601.

Khidr A (2003) Effects of the "Smith Accent Technique" of voice therapy on the laryngeal functions and voice quality of patients with unilateral vocal fold paralysis. *International Congress Series: Oto-Rhino-Laryngology. Proceedings of the XVII World Congress of the International Federation of Oto-Rhino-Laryngological Societies* (IFOS) 1240: 1235–1241. doi: http://dx.doi.org/10.1016/S0531-5131(03)00836-7

Mattioli F, Menichetti M, Bergamini G *et al.* (2015). Results of early versus intermediate or delayed voice therapy in patients with unilateral vocal fold paralysis: our experience in 171 patients *Journal of Voice* 29(4): 455–458. doi: 10.1016/j.jvoice.2014.09.027

Mattioli F, Bergamini G, Alicandri-Ciufelli M *et al.* (2011) The role of early voice therapy in the incidence of motility recovery in unilateral vocal fold paralysis Logopedics Phoniatrics Vocology 36(1): 40–47 doi: 10.3109/14015439.2011.554433

McFarlane SC, Holt-Romeo TL, Lavorato AS, Warne L (1991) Unilateral vocal fold paralysis: perceived vocal quality following three methods of treatment *American Journal of Speech-Language Pathology* 1(1): 45–48. doi: 10.1044/1058-0360.0101.45

NHMRC (1999) How to review the evidence: Systematic identification and review of scientific literature. Canberra, ACT: National Health and Medical Research Council Available at: http://www.nhmrc.gov.au/_files_nhmrc/publications/attachments/cp65.pdf [Accessed July 2016]

Paniello RC, Edgar JD, Kallogjeri D, Piccirillo JF (2011) Medialization versus reinnervation for unilateral vocal fold paralysis: a multicenter randomized clinical trial. *Laryngoscope* **121**(10): 2172–2179. doi: 10.1002/lary.21754

Ramig LO, Verdolini K (1998) Treatment efficacy: voice disorders *Journal of Speech, Language and Hearing Research* **41**(1): S101–S116. doi: 10.1044/jslhr.4101.s101

Rickert SM, Childs LF, Carey BT *et al.* (2012) Laryngeal electromyography for prognosis of vocal fold palsy: a meta-analysis *Laryngoscope* **122**(1): 158–161. doi: 10.1002/lary.22354

Robey RR (2004) A five-phase model for clinical-outcome research *Journal of Communication Disorders* **37**(5): 401–411. doi: 10.1016/j.jcomdis.2004.04.003

Schindler A, Bottero A, Capaccio P *et al.* (2008) Vocal improvement after voice therapy in unilateral vocal fold paralysis *Journal of Voice* **22**(1): 113–118. doi: 10.1016/j.jvoice.2006.08.004

Seyed Toutounchi SJ, Eydi M, Golzari SE *et al.* (2014) Vocal cord paralysis and its etiologies: a prospective study *Journal of Cardiovascular and Thoracic Research* **6**(1): 47–50. doi: 10.5681/jcvtr.2014.009

Sittel C, Stennert E, Thumfart WF *et al.* (2001) Prognostic value of laryngeal electromyography in vocal fold paralysis *Archives of Otolaryngology–Head & Neck Surgery* **127**(2): 155–160. doi: 10.1001/archotol.127.2.155

Spector BC, Netterville JL, Billante C *et al.* (2001) Quality-of-life assessment in patients with unilateral vocal cord paralysis *Otolaryngology–Head & Neck Surgery* **125**(3): 176–182.

Sulica L. (2008) The natural history of idiopathic unilateral vocal fold paralysis: evidence and problems *Laryngoscope* **118**(7): 1303–1307. doi: 10.1097/MLG.0b013e31816f27ee

Woodson G (2008) Evolving concepts of laryngeal paralysis *Journal of Laryngology and Otology* **122**(5): 437–441. doi: 10.1017/s002221510700045x

Zealear DL, Billante CR (2004) Neurophysiology of vocal fold paralysis *Otolaryngology Clinics of North America* **37**(1): 1–23.

# 7

# The effectiveness of voice therapy for Parkinson's disease-related voice disorder

## Patricia Gillivan-Murphy and Paul Carding

## Introduction

### Disease characteristics

Idiopathic Parkinson's disease (PD) is a progressive neurodegenerative disorder affecting approximately 1.5% of the population, or 7 million people worldwide (Pringsheim et al., 2014). The average age for the onset of PD is 59 years (Jankovic et al., 2001) but when it occurs in young people it is termed early onset PD (Jankovic et al., 2001) . The cardinal motor symptoms of PD are tremor, rigidity, akinesia and postural instability (Jankovic et al., 2008) which are related to the depletion of dopaminergic neurons in the substantia nigra pars compacta in the basal ganglia (Bergman et al., 2002). However, there are additional brain circuits involved in the disease process leading to a range of motor and sensory symptoms (Langston 2006). There is increasing awareness that PD is a multi-system disorder with symptoms of depression, anxiety, cognitive impairment and sensory impairment contributing to a complex clinical presentation (Braak et al., 2004).

Disease duration is generally measured from the time of clinical diagnosis and disease severity and there are important markers of PD disease. The Hoehn and Yahr scale (1967) is the most commonly used instrument for evaluating overall severity of PD, using a simple staging approach, ranging from stage 0 (no sign of disease) to stage 5 (wheelchair bound). Parts II and III of the Unified Parkinson's Disease Rating Scale (UPDRS) (Fahn *et al.*, 1987) are widely used clinically and include patient self-rating of activities of daily living and a clinician rating of motor signs respectively. It is important in PD voice treatment studies that authors report indices of disease severity. A specific treatment approach, for example, may work for patients with mild disease severity but may not be effective in a cohort of patients with greater severity of symptoms.

The mainstay treatment of the cardinal motor symptoms in PD is medication using dopamine replacement levodopa (L-dopa) which is converted to dopamine and dopamine agonists which directly stimulate dopamine receptors in the brain (Tolosa *et al.*, 2007). The positive effect of L-dopa on the limb symptoms of tremor, rigidity and akinesia is strongly established (Tolosa *et al.*, 2007). The effects of dopamine on speech and voice symptoms are unclear and variable (Schulz and Grant, 2000). For example, some studies show no effect while others show positive and negative effects of dopaminergic medication on speech and voice symptomatology (Spencer *et al.*, 2009; De Letter *et al.*, 2007; Goberman and Blomgren, 2003). Patients taking dopaminergic medication often experience cyclic fluctuations of their symptoms, with the term "on medication" used when motor symptoms are relieved and "off medication" when motor symptoms are present (Langston *et al.*, 1992). Medication status therefore is a possible confounder in speech and voice treatment studies and thus, it is important for studies to state whether patients are on a medication schedule and whether they are in an "on" or "off" state when assessment is carried out.

Deep Brain Stimulation (DBS) into the subthalamic nucleus (STN) is considered an effective treatment for those particular patients who develop dyskinesias from long term use of dopaminergic medication (Hammer *et al.*, 2010). However, the effects of DBS on speech and voice in patients with PD have been found to be variable or even adverse. For example, studies have reported excessive vocal fold closure (Hammer *et al.*, 2010), a reduction in glottic tremor (Klostermann *et al.*, 2008), increased vowel duration (Logemann and Fisher, 1981) and deterioration in speech intelligibility (Putzer *et al.*, 2008) with the stimulator switched on. Thus, it is again important for PD studies to indicate whether patients had received DBS pre-voice treatment and whether the stimulator was switched on or off when the outcome measures were collected.

## Speech and voice problems in PD

Motor speech and voice problems are strongly associated with PD (Logemann et al., 1981; Miller et al., 2007; Sapir et al., 2001) and severity is strongly related to disease progress (Sapir et al., 2001). The most frequently described perceptual speech and voice symptoms include low volume voice (hypophonia), breathiness, harsh voice quality, weak or asthenic voice, monopitch and monoloudness (prosodic disturbance), voice tremor, articulatory imprecision and variable rate of speech (Logemann et al., 1981; Miller et al., 2007; Sapir et al., 2001). This cluster of motor speech symptoms commonly known as hypokinetic dysarthria (Darley et al., 1975) occurs in more than 75% of people with PD (Logemann et al., 1978). There is consensus however that the voice-related features are central among the diverse symptomatology with voice impairment occurring more frequently than the other symptoms and featuring early in the disease process (Logemann et al., 1981; Miller et al., 2007; Stewart et al., 1995; Harel et al., 2004; Ho et al., 1998). Pathophysiological findings include bowing of the vocal folds (Hanson et al., 1984; Constantinescu et al., 2011), reduced activation of the thyroarytenoid muscles (Smith et al., 1995), tremor in the larynx (Carmichael et al., 2009) and weakness of the respiratory muscles (Carmichael et al., 2009). Speech and voice changes may lead to reduced speech intelligibility, which in turn impacts negatively on a person's communicative interaction and quality of life. Patients with PD have been shown to have increased voice disability when compared with neurologically healthy controls (Carmichael et al., 2009; Midi et al., 2008). For some patients, the speech and voice symptoms may be more problematic in daily living than the limb motor symptoms (Miller et al., 2008; Fox et al., 2002).

In addition to the myriad speech and voice symptoms, PD is associated with reduced facial expression (Jankovic, 2008), anxiety (Marinus et al., 2002), depression (Schrag, 2006) and cognitive impairment (Pillon et al., 1989; Sinforiani et al., 2008) and this contributes further to communicative disability. Patients with PD vary greatly both in clinical presentation and in the severity of symptoms regardless of the duration of the disease (Stewart et al., 1995; Metter and Hanson 1986; Chenery et al., 1988). Clinical heterogeneity contributes further to a complex clinical presentation. There is a strong positive correlation between PD and ageing (Van Den Eeden et al., 2003). It is expected that with changing demographics relating to an ageing population, speech and language therapists will be increasingly required to rehabilitate voice difficulties in people with PD. Therefore, knowledge of the effectiveness of voice therapy for PD is relevant and timely.

## General principles of treatment

Understanding of the underlying speech/voice pathophysiology in PD has increased in tandem with a range of developments including; new and improved methods of evaluation (laryngeal imaging, acoustic analysis, kinematics), easier access to brain imaging, greater understanding of principles of motor learning and relevance to speech and voice, knowledge of the effects of exercise on brain function (neuoroplasticity) and findings from studies using animal models. Improved knowledge and understanding of the core speech and voice pathophysiology has shaped treatment approaches for patients with PD.

Lowered sound pressure level (SPL dB), together with difficulty in calibrating and self-regulating levels of loudness, is considered to be a major contributory factor in the communicative problems of people with PD (Ramig *et al.*, 2001a). Understandably, therefore, treatments have focussed on increasing loudness in sustained vowel phonation and speech related contexts, i.e., reading aloud, picture description and monologue during conversation. Speech/voice therapy for patients with PD is essentially concerned with maximising speech/voice output to improve speech intelligibility.

## Searching the literature

For the purpose of writing this chapter, a literature search was carried out to identify relevant papers published between 2005 and 2015. Key words relating to Parkinson's disease, speech therapy, voice disorders and voice therapy were used to search different databases with the search limited to the English language. The initial search yielded 157 articles. The abstracts were reviewed and irrelevant articles were withdrawn, leaving a total of 44 studies. These 44 studies were reviewed for their relevance to the current chapter, namely studies that had behavioural voice-related treatment as a main focus of the study. Fifteen studies (Table 1) satisfied the criteria and their findings are analysed and interpreted in the following subsections.

Table 1: A Summary Of All Identified Relevant Studies

| Authors | n | Study Design | Type of Treatment | Outcome Measures | Findings |
|---|---|---|---|---|---|
| Theodoros et al., 2006 | 10 | Single arm | LSVT (web-based) | SPL sustained phonation, reading and monologue<br>Mean pitch range (Hz)<br>Perceptual ratings of 7 speech & voice variables on 5-point scale (speech intelligibility, articulatory precision, breathiness, hoarseness, pitch variability, loudness variability, loudness level) | Pre- vs. post-treatment differences<br>SPL all tasks $p < .0001$<br>Pitch range $p < 0.05$<br>Perceptual breathiness $p = 0.011$; pitch variability $p = 0.005$; loudness variability $p = 0.008$; loudness level $p < 0.01$.<br>Speech intelligibility, articulatory precision and hoarseness not significant |
| Sapir et al., 2007 | 44<br>14 = PD treatment<br>15 = PD no treatment<br>15 = controls | Randomised controlled trial | LSVT | SPL vowels /i/, /u/, /a/<br>Spectography F2u; F2i/F2u<br>Perceptual vowel rating (vowel goodness) /i/, /u/, /a/<br>Measures based on 3 read sentences | Pre vs. post treatment differences<br>In PD-T group<br>SPL vowels increased $p < .0001$<br>F2u $p < .0001$; F2i/F2u $p < .0001$<br>Vowel goodness improved $p = .0007$<br>In PD-NT and controls; no significant change in any measure |
| Spielman et al., 2007 | 12 | Single arm | LSVT (extended) | SPL sustained vowels and speech tasks<br>VHI | Pre- vs. post-treatment differences<br>SPL increased for all tasks $p < .001$<br>VHI scores reduced $p = 0.07$ |

| Authors | n | Study Design | Type of Treatment | Outcome Measures | Findings |
|---|---|---|---|---|---|
| Whitehill et al., 2007 | 4 | Case series | LSVT | Intonation sentence (perceptual rating VAS and paired comparison) SDF0 in sentence Lexical tone | Pre- vs post-treatment differences Intonation 4/4 subjects rated as less monotonous (VAS) Better intonation over 80% of time each subject SDF0 increased for 4/4 subjects No change in lexical tone for 4/4 subjects |
| Tindall et al., 2008 | 24 | Single arm study | LSVT (videophone) | SPL (sustained phonation and speech tasks) | Pre- vs post-treatment differences $P<0.01$ for all tasks |
| Di Bendetto et al., 2009 | 20 | Single arm study | Voice therapy & choral singing | *Respiratory function* Functional Residual Capacity (FRC%) Maximum Inspiratory Pressure (MIP) Maximum Expiratory Pressure (MEP) Forced vital capacity (FVC%) Forced Expiratory Volume 1 sec (FEV1%) Maximum duration sustained vowel phonation [71] *Acoustic voice measures (MDVP)* F0, vF0%, Jitter%, Shimmer %, vAm%, FTRI%, ATRI% *Auditory perceptual voice* Prosodia reading & monologue (10 cm VAS) Fatigue reading & monologue (Yes/No) | Pre- vs. post-treatment differences *Respiratory:* FRC%, MIP, MEP, MPT: ($p \leq 0.05$); FVC%, FEV1%: not significant *Acoustic:* none significant *Auditory perceptual* Prosodia reading: $p=0.046$ Prosodia monologue: not significant Fatigue reading: $p=0.05$ Fatigue monologue: not significant |

| Authors | n | Study Design | Type of Treatment | Outcome Measures | Findings |
|---|---|---|---|---|---|
| Howell et al., 2009 | 3 | Case series | LSVT (web & face-to-face combined) | SPL (sustained phonation & speech tasks)<br>Pitch (measured with a chromatic tuner)<br>Duration of sustained phonation (measured with a stop watch) | Pre- vs. post-treatment differences SPL increased for 3/3 subjects (ANOVA $p=0.01$)<br>Pitch not reported<br>Duration not reported |
| Constantinescu et al., 2011 | 34<br>17 = online LSVT 17 = face-to-face LSVT | Randomised controlled trial | LSVT (web) | SPL monologue<br>Vowel duration<br>Max fundamental frequency range<br>Perceptual voice parameters,<br>Intelligibility (word, sentences and overall speech)<br>Overall articulatory precision | 1. Online vs face-to-face treatment Non-inferiority of online LSVT confirmed for SPL monologue<br>2. Pre- vs post-treatment differences for online and face-to-face treatment SPL & max fundamental frequency range: ($p$ <0.05)<br>Vowel duration: no significant change<br>Perceptual voice parameters, word & sentence intelligibility & overall speech intelligibility: ($p$ <0.5)<br>Overall articulatory precision: no significant change |

| Authors | n | Study Design | Type of Treatment | Outcome Measures | Findings |
|---|---|---|---|---|---|
| Constantinescu et al, 2010 | 1 | Case study | LSVT (web) | SPL (sustained phonation & speech)<br>Vowel duration<br>Pitch range (semitones)<br>Perceptual voice rating (Direct Magnitude Estimate) for breathiness, roughness, loudness level, loudness & pitch variability, articulatory precision<br>speech intelligibility (conversation) | Pre- vs post-treatment differences<br>Increase in SPL for all tasks<br>Increase in MPT<br>No change in pitch range<br>Perceptual breathiness, roughness & overall speech intelligibility showed improvement<br>Articulatory precision: no change |
| Constantinescu et al, 2011 | 34<br>17 = online LSVT 17 = face-to-face LSVT | Randomised controlled trial | LSVT (web) | SPL monologue<br>Vowel duration<br>Max fundamental frequency range<br>Perceptual voice parameters,<br>Intelligibility (word, sentences and overall speech)<br>Overall articulatory precision | 1. Online vs face-to-face treatment<br>Non-inferiority of online LSVT confirmed for SPL monologue<br>2. Pre- vs post-treatment differences for online and face-to-face treatment<br>SPL & max fundamental frequency range: ($p$ <0.05)<br>Vowel duration: no significant change<br>Perceptual voice parameters, word & sentence intelligibility & overall speech intelligibility: ($p$ <0.5)<br>Overall articulatory precision: no significant change |

| Authors | n | Study Design | Type of Treatment | Outcome Measures | Findings |
|---|---|---|---|---|---|
| Whitehill et al., 2011 | 12 | Single arm | LSVT | Perceptual monotone (30 second reading task) using VAS<br>Perceptual lexical tone (tone transcription; tone error)<br>Acoustic SDF0 | Pre- vs post-treatment differences<br>Monotone: reduced ($p < 0.5$)<br>Lexical tone: no significant change<br>Mean SDF0 semitones: ($p = 0.9$), 4 subjects showed increase |
| Cannito et al., 2012 | 8 | Single arm | LSVT | SPL (vowels)<br>Perceived Intelligibility sentences (%) | Pre- vs post-treatment differences<br>Increased SPL vowels ($p = 0.003$)<br>% words understood increased ($p = 0.0001$)<br>(6/8 improved, 1 deteriorated, 1 = no change in intelligibility |
| Halpern et al., 2012 | 16<br>8 = PD immediate treatment<br>8 = PD delayed treatment | Randomised controlled trial | LSVT combined (face-to-face) and assistive technology (LSVT Companion) | SPL (sustained vowel and varied speech tasks)<br>Perceptual rating of sentence pairs on global voice and speech parameters (much better/much worse)<br>VHI<br>Ratings by significant other (SO) (VAS) and Modified Communicative Effectiveness Index (CETI-M)<br>Ratings (1–5) of "helpfulness" of Companion by participants & SO | Pre- vs post-treatment differences<br>SPL: increased across tasks ($p < .0001$)<br>Perceptual rating: significant difference ($p < .0001$)<br>VHI: no significant change post-treatment or follow up<br>SO VAS: significant change ($p < .05$) for monotone, hoarseness, loudness, speaks to be understood<br>SO CETI-M: total rating significant change ($p < .01$) for travelling in car, noisy environment, long conversation<br>13/16 subjects rated Companion as "5"(very helpful)<br>10/13 SO rated Companion as "5" |

| Authors | n | Study Design | Type of Treatment | Outcome Measures | Findings |
|---|---|---|---|---|---|
| Shih et al., 2012 | 13 | Single arm | Choral singing (group) | SPL (reading aloud)<br>VHI<br>VRQOL | Pre- vs post-treatment differences<br>Non significant for<br>SPL<br>VHI<br>VRQOL |
| Sauvageau et al., 2015 | 9 | Single arm | LSVT | SPL (sustained phonation & speech tasks)<br>Acoustic formant frequencies (/i/, u/, /a/) in reading;<br>Acoustic vowel space (AVS) (Hz);<br>Vowel SPL ;<br>Vowel duration;<br>Consonant vowel (C-V) coarticulation | Pre- vs post-treatment differences<br>SPL increased $p<0.001$ (for all 4 tasks)<br>AVS increased $p<0.05$<br>Vowel SPL increased $p<0.001$<br>Vowel duration increased $p<0.001$<br>C-V coarticulation significant change ($p<0.001$) |
| Sale et al., 2015 | 39<br>PD (23) PSP (16) | Double arm<br>PD group<br>PSP group | LSVT | 14 different measures<br>High frequencies (Hz) maximum and mean Low frequencies (Hz) minimum and mean Sustained /a/ (dB) minimum and maximum Sustained /a/ durations (sec's) minimum and maximum<br>Sentence, reading, speaking (dB) minimum and maximum | Pre- vs post-treatment differences<br>PD group<br>11 measures significant change $p$ values ($p<0.05$)<br>PSP group<br>7 measures significant change $p$ values $p<0.05$<br>Difference between PD & PSP groups post treatment: no difference across 14 measures ($p>0.05$) |

## Systematic reviews of speech/voice therapy efficacy

There are two Cochrane reviews relevant to this chapter and both were published in 2012. The first Cochrane review included all randomised controlled trials (RCTs) that compared a defined speech/voice therapy technique with a placebo or no intervention group (Herd et al., 2012a). Herd et al. (2012a) identified three relevant trials (Robertson and Thomson, 1984; Johnson and Pring, 1990; Ramig et al., 2001b), but these studies are not included in the summary of recent relevant treatment efficacy studies in PD in Table 1, because they were published before 2005. The authors of this systematic review identified a number of key methodological problems which included: an insufficient number of participants in the trials (which can lead to selection bias and false positive or false negative conclusions); the methods of randomisation were either not reported or inappropriately administered; the eligibility criteria were not clearly stated (for example the diagnostic criteria or disease severity rating were not defined); and inclusion/exclusion criteria were not stated. Herd et al., (2012a) concluded that there was insufficient evidence to conclusively support or refute the efficacy of speech/voice therapy for patients with PD and recommended that further large, well-designed placebo-controlled RCTs were necessary to assess the effectiveness of speech and language therapy for speech disorders in PD.

The second Cochrane Collaboration Systematic review, also carried out by Herd et al., (2012b), compared different speech/voice therapy techniques for speech/voice problems in PD. This systematic review included all randomised controlled trials (RCTs) that compared two types of speech/voice therapy in an individual study. In total, six studies were identified as appropriate for inclusion. A number of different treatment techniques were compared including prosodic exercise techniques with visual feedback, LSVT vs respiratory therapy, LSVT LOUD vs modified LSVT, methods of delivery of LSVT and rate reduction techniques (Scott and Caird, 1983; Baumgartner et al., 2001; Healy, 2002; Halpern et al., 2012; Lowitt et al., 2010; Constantinescu et al., 2011). Studies carried out by Halpern et al., (2012) and Constantinescu et al., (2011) are included in the summary in Table 1 of relevant recent published studies of treatment efficacy. The study by Lowit et al., (2010) is not included in the Table because it did not include behavioural voice treatment as one of its main treatment approaches. This study did, however, examine the effectiveness of delayed auditory feedback using a device versus traditional speech therapy to reduce speech rate and improve speech intelligibility. The authors of the systematic review (Herd et al., 2012b) concluded that there was insufficient evidence to support or refute the efficacy of any form of SLT over another to treat speech/voice problems in patients with

PD. The methodological weaknesses of the published RCTs had a significant bearing on the quality and trustworthiness of the published results. This second review also included a number of recommendations to improve the quality and nature of the evidence of voice therapy efficacy for patients with PD (Herd et al., 2012b). The most common and significant methodological shortcomings identified are as follows:

(a) The lack of firm and clear diagnostic criteria
(b) The small numbers of study participants which may lead to false negative or false positive conclusions
(c) Non-uniformity of patient cohorts (i.e. disease onset, severity and presentation)
(d) The lack of follow-up beyond the immediate end of treatment
(e) Lack of clarity about "on" versus "off" medication/treatment state.

Two Level II randomised controlled studies have been carried out since these systematic reviews and are within the relevant time period of 2005–2015 (Sapir et al., 2007; Constantinescu 201) for the purpose of this chapter. Both studies used Lee Silverman Voice Treatment (LSVT) as the treatment approach. Sapir et al., (2007) examined the effects of LSVT on vowel articulation in a group of patients with PD randomised to a treatment and a no-treatment group. They also studied an age matched healthy control group. Importantly, they found that there was no significant differences between the treatment and no-treatment group post randomisation on variables of age, number of years since diagnosis, stage of disease, or severity of speech and voice disorder prior to treatment. However, the method of randomisation was not reported in the study. A range of vowel related measures was used including: vowel sound pressure level (SPL); various features of the first (F1) and second (F2) formants of the vowels /i/,/u/,/a/; vowel triangle area; perceptual vowel ratings. The authors reported that there were significant changes in the PD group treated with LSVT in the following measures: SPL vowels; F2 of the vowel /u/ (F2u); the ratio of F2 of vowel /i/ (F2i) to F2 of vowel /u/ (F2u); and perceptual rating of vowel goodness. The authors concluded that increased loudness improves vowel articulation in patients with PD treated with LSVT. Outcome measures were collected at the immediate post treatment time only, therefore further studies are required to determine if LSVT has longer term effects on vowel articulation. It is worthy of note that the positive treatment outcome was based on three read aloud sentences and not spontaneous speech. However, while a recording of conversational speech may be preferable, it is acknowledged that this is a more difficult context to control for assessment purposes.

Constantinescu et al. (2011) studied the validity and reliability of LSVT delivered either online or face-to-face in a group of 34 patients with PD. First, the PD group were stratified based on dysarthria severity classification and subsequently randomised to either the LSVT face-to-face or to online treatment. The randomisation method was carried out using a computerised random-number generator. The study findings showed that LSVT delivered online was not inferior to LSVT delivered face-to-face on the primary outcome measure of SPL in a monologue task. There were significant treatment effects from LSVT delivered online or face-to-face for a range of measures including SPL, maximum fundamental frequency range, perceptual voice measures and speech intelligibility. In contrast duration of vowel phonation showed little change post-LSVT (in both treatment groups). The measures were collected immediately post treatment only and therefore it is unknown whether the treatment effects were maintained over time.

## Recent (non RCT) studies of LSVT efficacy

Most of the treatment studies reviewed for this chapter may be categorised as Level III evidence or lower (Sauvageau et al., 2015; Theodoros et al., 2006; Spielman et al., 2007; Whitehill and Wong, 2007; Di Benedetto et al., 2009; Tindall et al., 2008; Howell et al., 2009; Constantinescu et al., 2010; Whitehill et al., 2011; Cannito et al., 2012; Shih et al., 2012). The numbers of patients treated in any single study were small and ranged from one patient in a single case study (Constantinescu et al., 2010) to a maximum of 24 patients in a single arm study (Tindall et al., 2008). Minimising potential sources of bias is an important aspect to control in treatment studies. One possible source of bias relates to the manner in which participants are recruited to a study. Several of these Level III studies did not report on the manner in which participants were recruited (Theodoros et al., 2006; Spielman et al., 2007; Whitehill and Wong, 2007; Tindall et al., 2008; Whitehill et al., 2011; Shih et al., 2012).

Generally, patients were evaluated and treated while on a stable dopaminergic medication regime. Two studies reported that patients were taking medication but the authors did not state whether the regime was constant throughout the study (Constantinescu et al., 2011; Whitehill and Wong, 2007) and three studies did not provide any information on medication status for their patients (Theodoros et al., 2006; Tindall et al., 2008; Shih et al., 2012).

## Treatment approaches

The majority of studies reviewed used the Lee Silverman Voice Treatment (LSVT®) (Ramig *et al.*, 1994) method or variants thereof. The two non-LSVT treatment studies used a combined voice and choral singing approach (Whitehill and Wong, 2007) or choral singing as a stand-alone treatment (Shi *et al.*, 2012).

### Lee Silverman Voice Treatment (LSVT)

The Lee Silverman Voice Treatment (LSVT®) method was developed to treat the core problem of hyopophonia in patients with PD (Ramig *et al.*, 1994). It is an intensive behavioural treatment that focuses on a simple target of "think loud" and is delivered in four 50-minute sessions over a consecutive four-week period totalling 16 sessions. LSVT promotes increased respiratory drive, vocal fold adduction and increased vocal loudness in everyday communication (Ramig *et al.*, 1994). In addition to the positive effects on the core problem of low volume voice, there are claims that LSVT may have wider speech and voice benefits, including increasing facial expression, jaw opening and improved articulation (Ramig *et al.*, 1996; Ramig *et al.*, 2001b; Ramig *et al.*, 1994). This review of recent studies shows that patients are receiving LSVT in different modes and with variation on the standard (prescribed) 16 sessions.

Studies have delivered LSVT face-to face (Sapir *et al.*, 2007; Whitehill and Wong 2007; Whitehill *et al.*, 2011; Cannito *et al.*, 2012; Sale *et al.*, 2015), via web cam (Constantinescu *et al.*, 2011; Theodoros *et al.*, 2006; Tindal *et al.*, 2008; Constantinescu *et al.*, 2010), combined web cam and face-to face (Howell *et al.*, 2009) and combined face-to-face with assistive technology (LSVT ® Companion) (Halpern *et al.*, 2012). The development of different modes of delivery reflects the increasing difficulty that clinicians are encountering in delivering 16 face-to face treatment sessions over a four-week period. Difficulties relate to time investment, costs and in some cases geographical distances between clinicians and patients. Most of the LSVT studies followed the standard 16 sessions delivered over a four-week period. In contrast, two studies (Spielman *et al.*, 2007; de Azevedo *et al.*, 2015) used an "extended" version of LSVT whereby the patient receives 16 sessions in an eight-week rather than a four-week period. The "extended" version of LSVT is designed to lessen the burden on the patient and the clinician.

# Treatment outcomes

## Sound pressure level

An increase in sound pressure level (SPL) has been the focus of most of the treatment studies using LSVT. It is of note that all of the studies reported significant increases in SPL across different contexts, i.e., vowels, reading and monologue. Importantly, from a service delivery perspective, the gains in SPL were broadly similar regardless of whether treatment was delivered face-to-face (Spielman et al., 2007; Cannito et al., 2012; Suavageau et al., 2015), remotely (Theodoros et al., 2006; Constantinescu et al., 2010) or with a combined face-to-face and remote approach (Howell et al., 2009).

## Speech intelligibility and communication effectiveness

An overarching goal of voice therapy in PD is to improve speech intelligibility and communicative effectiveness. Studies that addressed speech intelligibility and communication outcomes were all LSVT based and reported positive findings across different speaking contexts (Theodoros et al., 2006; Constantinescu et al., 2010; Constantinescu et al., 2011; Cannito et al., 2012). In a study of 10 patients using web-based LSVT Theodoros et al. (2006) reported a trend to improvement in mean scores post-treatment in reading aloud and conversational monologue tasks. Also using web-based LSVT, Constantinescu et al., (2010) in a single case study identified improvement in overall speech intelligibility based on a 30 second conversation monologue. Constantinescu et al. (2011) in a non-inferiority trial of 34 patients randomised to receiving either face-to-face or web-based LSVT, found significant improvement in word, sentence and overall speech intelligibility in both groups. Cannito et al., (2012) found that there was a significant difference post-LSVT in a group of eight patients when measured on the percentage of words understood in sentences. It is important to note that six patients showed improvement, one deteriorated and one showed no change in intelligibility (Cannito et al., 2012). Furthermore, in a study of 16 patients receiving combined LSVT with the LSVT companion (interactive technology), Halpern et al., (2012) reported significant changes in the all patients' speech intelligibility and communication effectiveness as judged by their partner or carer.

## Voice disability

The effect of voice treatment on patient reported voice disability shows mixed findings. Three studies examined the effects of voice treatment on patient-reported voice disability (Halpern *et al.*, 2012; Spielman *et al.*, 2007; Shih *et al.*, 2012). Halpern *et al.*, (2012), using LSVT, found that mean scores on the Voice Handicap Index (VHI) (Jacobsen *et al.*, 1997) reduced from 45 to 31. For an individual patient, a reduction of this magnitude would be considered clinically significant, although the mean change for the study group was not statistically significant. Spielman *et al.*, 2007) also using LSVT reported a lowering of mean group VHI scores from 44 to 31 without statistical significance. However, they found that 4 out of 12 patients (33%) showed significant improvements, with each person lowering his/her score by 31 points or more. Finally, Shih *et al.*, (2012), in a study using group choral singing, reported an increase (deterioration) in mean VHI scores from 43 to 47. Patients with PD have variable clinical presentation and varied treatment outcomes. It is important to remember that individual treatment effects (benefits or risks) may not be captured by group data and it is therefore also important for studies to provide outcome data from individual patients in addition to group data.

## Laryngeal and vocal fold function

A fundamental tenet of the LSVT treatment approach is that the loud voicing with increased effort improves vocal fold adduction and sound pressure level. It is acknowledged that there is a risk of patients developing secondary laryngeal hyperfunction (Ramig *et al.*, 1994). The majority of studies reviewed reported that laryngeal examination was carried out to exclude laryngeal pathology prior to LSVT. Of note, however, is that none of the LSVT-based studies reported treatment outcomes on laryngeal function or vocal fold closure patterns. Therefore there is no knowledge of whether LSVT induced laryngeal hyperfunction or not. In contrast, Di Bendetto *et al.*, (2009) in a pilot study of 20 patients with PD treated with speech therapy and choral singing, evaluated a range of stroboscopic features including symmetry of vocal fold movement, amplitude of movement and glottic closure (Di Benedetto *et al.*, 2009). They stated that the post-treatment videostroboscopy results were the same for each individual patient. However, they did not furnish data on specific findings, their method of evaluating the laryngeal examinations and/or reliability of data interpretation.

## Timing of outcome measurement

An issue occurs when interpreting treatment outcome if a study does not report the time interval between the end of treatment and the collection of outcome measures (Constantinescu, 2010; Shih et al., 2012; Theodoros et al., 2006). Studies show great variability in relation to the time that outcome data is collected relative to the end of treatment. For example, post-treatment outcomes were collected immediately after the treatment programme in some studies (Constantinescu et al., 2011; Sapir et al., 2007) and within a one to two-week (Whitehill and Wong 2007; Di Benedetto et al., 2009; Tindal et al., 2008; Cannito et al., 2012) and one to six-month period (Sauvageau et al., 2015; Howell et al., 2009; Shih et al., 2012) for other studies. Clinicians will be understandably more confident in a treatment approach that has been shown to be effective immediately after treatment and is maintained six months after treatment.

## Summary findings

This review of voice treatment effectiveness in patients with Parkinson's disease shows that the primary focus of voice treatment in the period 2005 to 2015 has been to increase vocal sound pressure level (SPL), in sustained phonation and speech tasks. The main treatment approach used has been the Lee Silverman Voice Treatment (LSVT) and this has been shown to increase SPL across a range of tasks. The increasing challenge faced by SLT's in delivering 16 sessions of face-to-face LSVT over a four-week period is reflected in the literature, with studies reporting on remotely delivered LSVT and combined LSVT approaches.

A number of issues and areas for development have emerged from the treatment studies reviewed.

- Outcome measures should be collected at least six months after the completion of treatment to evaluate the long term effectiveness of treatment and assist clinicians in decision making regarding treatment.
- Rating laryngeal features for example, vocal fold bowing, vocal fold closure patterns, vocal tract tremor and supra-glottic constriction pre- and post-treatment would improve knowledge of laryngeal pathophysiology in patients with PD and the effect that voice therapy has on laryngeal function.
- Greater attention to the effect of increased SPL on communication effectiveness in voice treatment studies is warranted. Therefore, studies should include measures that address the views of a patient's "significant other" in relation to a patient's communication effectiveness.

## References

Baumgartner C, Sapir S, Ramig L. Perceptual voice quality changes following phonatory-respiratory effort treatment (LSVT) vs respiratory effort treatment for individuals with Parkinson's disease. *Journal of Voice* 2001;**15**:105–14.

Bergman H, Deuschl G. Pathophysiology of Parkinson's Disease: From clinical neurology to basic neuroscience and back. *Movement Disorders* 2002;**17**(3):S28–S40.

Braak H, Ghebremehin E, Rub U, Bratzke H, Del Tredici K. Stages in the development of Parkinson's disease-related pathology. *Cell Tissue Research* 2004;**318**:121–34.

Cannito M, Suiter D, Beverly D, Chorna L, Wolf T, Pfeiffer R. Sentence intelligiblity before and after voice treatment in speakers with idiopathic Parkinson's disease. *Journal of Voice* 2012;**26**(2):214–19.

Carmichael C, Ruddy B. respiratory function & self perceived voice handicap in patient's with Parkinson's Disease. *Texas Journal of Audiology & Speech Language Pathology* 2009;**32**:35–45.

Chenery J, Murdoch B, Ingram J. Studies in Parkinson's Disease: 1. Perceptual speech analyses. *Australian Journal of Human Communication Disorders* 1988;**16**:17–29.

Constantinescu G, Theodoros D, Russell T, WArd E, Wilson S, Wooton R. Treating disordered speech and voice in Parkinson's disease online: a randomised controlled non-inferiority trial. *International journal of Language & Communication Disorders* 2011;**46**(1):1–16.

Constantinescu G, Theodoros D, Russell T, Ward E, Wilson S, Wooton R. Home-based speech treatment for Parkinson's disease delivered remotely: a case report. *Journal of Telemedicine and Telecare* 2010;**16**:100–04.

Darley F, Aronson A, Brown J. *Motor Speech Disorders*. Philadelphia: WB Saunders Company, 1975.

de Azevedo L, de Souze I, de Oliveira P, Cardoso F. Effect of speech therapy and pharmacological treatment in prosody of parkinsonians. *Arq Neuropsiquiatr* 2015;**73**(1):30–35.

De Letter M, Santens P, De Bodt M, Van Maele G, Van Borsel J, Boon P. The effect of levodopa on respiration and word intelligibility in people with advanced Parkinson's disease. *Clinical Neurology & Neuropsychiatry* 2007;**109**:495–500.

Deuschl G, Paschen S, Witt K. Clinical outcome of deep brain stimulation for Parkinson's disease. *Handbook of Clinical Neurology* 2013;**116**:107–28.

Di Benedetto P, Cavazzon M, Mondolo F, Rugiu G, Peratoner A, E B. Voice and choral singing treatment: a new approach for speech and voice disorders in Parkinson's disease. *European Journal of Physical & Rehabilitation Medicine* 2009;**45**:13–19.

Fahn S, Elton R. Unified Parkinson's Disease Rating Scale In: Fahn S, Goldstein M, D M, Calne D, editors. *Recent Developments in Parkinson's Disease*. New Jersey: Macmillan Healthcare Information, 1987:153–63.

Fox C, Morrison C, Ramig L, Shapir S. Current perspectives on the Lee Silverman Voice Treatment (LSVT) for individuals with idiopathic Parksinson Disease. *American Journal of Speech-Language Pathology* 2002;**11**:111–23.

Goberman A, Blomgren M. Parkinsonian speech dysfluencies: effects of L-dopa-related fluctuations. *Journal of Fluency Disorders* 2003;28:55–70.

Hammer M, Barlow S, Lyons K, Pahwa R. Subthalamic nucleus deep brain stimulation changes in speech respiratory and laryngeal control in Parkinson's disease. *Journal of Neurology* 2010;257:1692–702.

Hanson D, Gerratt B, Ward P. Cinegraphic observations of vocal pathology in Parkinson's disease. *Laryngoscope* 1984;92:348–53.

Harel B, Cannizzaro M, Cohen H, Reilly N, Snyder P. Acoustic characteristics of Parkinsonian speech: a potential biomarker of early disease progression and treatment. *Journal of Neurolinguistics* 2004;17:439–53.

Healy V. A comparison of the efficacy of two methods of rate control in the speech of people with Parkinson's disease. *Internal report, Manchester Royal Infirmary* 2002.

Herd CP, Tomlinson CL, Deane KHO, Brady MC, Smith CH, Sackley CM, *et al*. Comparison of speech and language therapy techniques for speech problems in Parkinson's disease. *Cochrane Database of Systematic Reviews* 2012a;8:1–69.

Herd CP, Tomlinson CL, Deane KHO, Brady MC, Smith CH, Sackley CM, *et al*. Speech and language therapy versus placebo or no intervention for speech problems in Parkinson's disease (Review). *Cochrane Database of Systematic Reviews* 2012b;8.

Ho A, Iansek R, Marigliania C, Bradshaw J, Gates S. Speech impairment in a large sample of patients with Parkinson's disease. *Behavioural Neurology* 1998;11:131–37.

Hoehn M, Yahr M. Parkinsonism:onset, progression and mortality. *Neurology* 1967;17:427–42.

Howell S, Tripoliti E, Pring T. Delivering the Lee Silverman Voice Treatment (LSVT) by web camera: a feasibility study. *International journal of Language & Communication Disorders* 2009;44(4):287–300.

Jacobsen B, Johnson A, Grywalski C, Silbergleit A, Jacobsen G, Beninger M. The Voice Handicap Index (VHI): Development and validation. *American Jounal of Speech & Language Pathology* 1997;6:66–70.

Jankovic J. Parkinson's disease: clinical features and diagnosis. *Journal of Neurology, Neurosurgery & Psychiatry* 2003;79:368–76.

Jankovic J. Functional decline in Parkinson's Disease. *Archives of Neurology* 2001;58:1611–15.

Jankovic J, Mc Dermott M, Carter J, Gauthier S, Goetz C, Golbe L, *et al*. Variable expression of Parkinson's disease: a base-line analysis of the DATATOP cohort- the Parkinson Study Group. *Neurology* 1990;40:1529–34.

Johnson JA, Pring TR. Speech therapy and Parkinson's disease: A review and further data. *British Journal of Disorders of Communication* 1990;25:183–94.

Klostermann F, Ehlen F, Vesper J, Nubel K, Gross M, Marzinzik F, *et al*. Effects of subthalmic deep brain stimulation on dysarthrophonia in Parkinson's disease. *Journal of Neurology, Neurosurgery & Psychiatry* 2008;79:522–29.

Langston J. The Parkinson's complex: Parkinsonism is just the tip of the iceberg. *Annals of Neurology* 2006;59(4):591–96.

Langston J, Widner H, Goetz C. Core Assessment Program for Intracerebral Transplantations. *Movement Disorders* 1992;7:2-13.

Lim A, LiPyn L, Huckabee M-L, Frampton C, Anderson T. A pilot study of respiration and swallowing integration in Parkinson's Disease: "On" and "off" levodopa. *Dysphagia* 2008;**23**:76–81.

Logemann J, Fisher H, Boshes B, Blonsky R. Frequency & co-occurrence of vocal tract dysfunctions in the speech of large sample of Parkinson patients. *Journal of Speech & Hearing Disorders* 1978;**43**:47–57.

Logemann J, Fisher H. Vocal tract control in Parkinson's disease. *Journal of Speech & Hearing Disorders* 1981;**46**:348–52.

Lowit A, Dobinson C, Timmins C, Howell P, Kroger B. The effectiveness of traditional methods and altered auditory feedback in improving speech rate and intelligibility in speakers with Parkinson's disease. *International Journal of Speech-Language Pathology* 2010;**12**(5):426–36.

Marinus J, Leentgens A, Visser M, Stigggelbout A, Van Hilten J. Evaluation of the hospital anxiety & depression scale in patients with Parkinson's Disease. *Clinical Neuropharmacology* 2002;**25**: 318–24.

Metter E, Hanson W. Clinical and acoustical variability in hypokinetic dysarthria. *Journal of Communication Disorders* 1986;**19**:347–66.

Midi I, Dogan M, Koseoglu M, Can G, Sehitoglu M, Gunal D. Voice abnormalities and their relation with motor dysfunction in Parkinson's disease. *Acta Neurological Scandinavia* 2008;**117**:26–34.

Miller N, Allcock L, Jones D, Burns D. How do I sound to me? Perceived changes in communication in Parkinson's disease *Clinical Rehabilitation* 2008;**22**(1):14.

Miller N, Allcock L, Jones D, Noble E, Hildreth A, Burn D. Prevalence and pattern of perceived intelligibility changes in Parkinson's disease. *Journal of Neurology, Neurosurgery & Psychiatry* 2007;**78**:1180–90.

Perez K, Ramig L, Smith M, Dromey C. The Parkinson larynx: tremor and videostroboscopic findings. *Journal of Voice* 1996;**10**(4):354–61.

Pillon B, Dubois B, Cusimano G, Bonnett A-M, Lhermitte F, Agid Y. Does cognitive impairment in Parkinson's disease result from non-dopaminergic lesions? *Journal of Neurology, Neurosurgery & Psychiatry* 1989;**52**:201–06.

Pringsheim T, Jette N, Frolkis A, Steeves T. The prevalence of Parkinson's disease: a systematic review and meta-analysis. *Movement Disorders* 2014;**29**(13):1583–90.

Pützer M, Barry W, Moringlane J. Effect of bilateral stimulation of the sub-thalamic nucleus on different speech subsystems inpatients with Parkinson's disease. *Clinical Linguistics and Phonetics* 2008;**22**:957–73.

Ramig L, Sapir S, Countryman S, Pawlas A, O'Brien C, Hoehn M, *et al*. Intensive voice treatment (LSVT ®) for patients with Parkinson's disease: a 2 year follow up. *Journal of Neurology, Neurosurgery and Psychiatry* 2001a;**71**:493–98.

Ramig LO, Sapir S, Fox C, Countryman S. Changes in vocal loudness following intensive voice treatment (LSVT®) in individuals with Parkinson's disease: A comparison with untreated patients and normal age-matched controls. *Movement Disorders* 2001b;**16**(1):79–83.

Ramig L, Countryman S, O'Brien C, Hoehn M, Thompson L. Intensive speech treatment for patients with Parkinson's disease: Short-and long-term comparison of two techniques. 1996.

Ramig LO, Bonitati CM, Lemke JH, Horri Y. Voice treatment for patients with Parkinson disease: development of an approach and preliminary efficacy data. *Journal of Medical Speech-Language Pathology* 1994;**2**:191–209.

Robertson SJ, Thomson F. Speech therapy in Parkinson's disease: a study of the efficacy and long term effects of intensive treatment. *British Journal of Disorders of Communication* 1984;**19**:213–24.

Sale P, Castiglioni D, De Pandis M, Torti M, Dallarmi V, Radicati G, et al. The Lee Silverman Voice Treatment (LSVT®) speech therapy in progressive supranuclear palsy. *European Journal of Physical & Rehabilitation Medicine* 2015;**51**(5).

Sapir S, Spielman J, Ramig L, Story B, Fox C. Effects of intensive voice treatment [the Lee Silverman Voice Treatment (LSVT)] on vowel articulation in dysarthric individuals with idiopathic Parkinson disease: acoustic and perceptual findings. [Erratum appears in *Journal Speech Language & Hearing Research* 2007 Dec; 50(6):1652]. *Journal of Speech, Language & Hearing Research* 2007;**50**(4):899912.

Sapir S, Pawlas A, Ramig L, Countryman S, O'Brien C, Hoehn M, et al. Voice and speech abnormalities in Parkinson disease: Relation to Severity of motor impairment, duration of disease, medication, depression, gender and age. *Journal of Medical Speech-Language Pathology* 2001;**9**(4):213–26.

Sauvageau V, Roy J-P, M L, J M. Impact of the LSVT on vowel articulation and coarticulation in Parkinson's disease. *Clinical Linguistics and Phonetics* 2015;**29**(6):424–40.

Schrag A. Quality of life and depression in Parkinson's Disease. *Journal of Neurological Science* 2006;**248**:151–57.

Schulz G, Grant M. Effects of speech therapy and pharmacologic and surgical treatments on voice and speech in Parkinson's disease: a review of the literature. *Journal of Communication Disorders* 2000;**33**:59–88.

Scott S, Caird FI. Speech therapy for Parkinson's disease. *Journal of Neurology, Neurosurgery and Psychiatry* 1983;**46**:140–4.

Shih L, Piel J, Warren A, Kraics L, Silver A, Vanderhorst V, et al. Singing in groups for Parkinson's disease (SING-PD): A pilot study of group singing therapy for PD-related voice/speech disorders. *Parkinsonism and Related Disorers* 2012;**18**:548–52.

Sinforiani E, Pacchetti C, Zangaglia R, Pasotti C, Manni R, Nappi KG. REM Behaviour disorder, hallucinations and cognitive impairment in Parkinson's Disease: A two-year follow up. *Movement Disorders* 2008;**23**(10):1441–45.

Smith M, Ramig L, Dromey C, Perez K. Intensive voice treatment in Parkinson's disease:laryngostroboscopic findings. *Journal of Voice* 1995;**9**:453–59.

Spencer K, Morgan K, Blond E. Dopaminergic medication effects on the speech of individuals with Parkinson's Disease. *Journal of Medical Speech-Language Pathology* 2009;**17**(3):125–44.

Spielman J, Ramig L, Mahler L, Halpern A, Gavin W. Effects of an extended version of the Lee Silverman Voice Treatment on voice and speech in Parkinson's Disease. *American Journal of Speech-Language Pathology* 2007;**16**(2):95–107.

Stewart C, Winfield L, Hunt A, Bressman S, Fahn S, Blitzer A, *et al.* Speech Dysfunction in Early Parkinson's Disease. *Movement Disorders* 1995;**10**(5):562–65.

Theodoros DG, Constantinescu G, Russell TG, Ward EC, Wilson SJ, Wootton R. Treating the speech disorder in Parkinson's disease online. *Journal of Telemedicine and Telecare* 2006;**12**(3):88–91.

Tindall L, Huebner R, Stemple J, Kleinert H. Videophone-delivered voice therapy: a comparative analysis of outcomes to traditional delivery for adults with Parkinson's Disease. *Telemedicine and e-Health* 2008;**14**(10):1070–77.

Tolosa E, Katzenschlager R. Pharmacological management of Parkinson's Disease. In: Jankovic J, Tolosa E, editors. *Parkinson's Disease & Movement Disorders*. 5 ed. Philadelphia: Lippincott Williams & Wilkins, 2007:110–45.

Van Den Eeden S, Tanner C, Bernstein A. Incidence of Parkinson's disease: variation by age, gender and race/ethnicity. *American Journal of Epidemiology* 2003;**157**:1015–22.

Whitehill T, Wong L. Effect of intensive voice treatment on tone-language speakers with Parkinson's disease. *Clinical Linguistics and Phonetics* 2007;**21**(11–12):919–25.

Whitehill TL, Kwan L, Lee FP, Chow MM. Effect of LSVT on lexical tone in speakers with Parkinson's Disease. *Parkinson's Disease* 2011:897494.

# 8

# Techniques for measuring voice outcomes of therapy interventions

## Paul Carding

### Choosing the most appropriate outcome measure

High quality study design of treatment effectiveness must include the careful and considered choice of the most appropriate outcome measures. The wrong and inappropriate choice of outcome measures can, at best, weaken the conclusions of a study and at worst, invalidate the study findings altogether. Olswang (1998) made an important observation, that outcomes can only be defined in terms of the agent. Thus, outcomes can be:

- Clinically-derived – for example, clinical measures such as maximum phonation time or perceptual rating of voice quality
- Functional – for example, a measure of how the patient is functioning in his/her work or social life
- Administrative – for example, activity data regarding the amount, frequency and duration of therapy sessions
- Financial – for example, a measure of the cost of a programme of voice therapy or the cost to the patient of not being able to work as a consequence of the voice disorder
- Client-defined – for example, the perceived improvement in quality of life or the rating of speaking confidence in a social setting.

The topic of this book is treatment effectiveness and hence, our focus remains upon clinically-derived, functional and client-defined techniques for measuring voice outcomes of therapy intervention.

It is important to make a distinction between clinical assessment tools and outcome measurement tools. The essential purposes of clinical assessment are to aid differential diagnosis, to understand the nature and impact of the disorder and to inform management decision making and treatment design. The essential purpose of outcome measurement is to quantify change over time. The possible confusion lies in the fact that some clinical assessment instruments can also be used as outcome measures (i.e., they can be used for two purposes). However, there are many assessment tools which would make very poor outcome measures for reasons that will be discussed below. Equally there are many voice outcome measures that may be of limited value in aiding differential diagnosis or helping to design voice therapy.

There is a large number of potential voice outcome measures to choose from. These can be divided into seven broad categories, as listed in the table below:

Table 1: The Seven Broad Categories of Voice Outcome Measurement Techniques

| Category of Outcome Measurement | Main Techniques |
| --- | --- |
| Aerodynamic measurements | Maximum phonation time, s/z ratio, subglottal pressure, glottal resistance, glottal efficiency, airflow intensity, airflow rate, phonation quotient, vocal velocity index, vital capacity, pulmonary function tests |
| Measurements of fundamental frequency and intensity | Fundamental frequency ($F_0$ range, speaking or habitual $F_0$, intensity range (or sound pressure level), speaking or habitual SPL, voice range profile (VRP/phonetograhy) |
| Visual perceptual measurements | Flexible endoscopy ratings, stroboscopy ratings, ultra-high speed photography |
| Auditory perceptual measurements | Perceptual ratings of voice quality |
| Physiological measurements | Laryngography (EGG), photoglottography, electromyography |
| Acoustic analysis of the sound waveform | Sound spectrogram, pitch perturbation, amplitude perturbation, signal to noise ratio, harmonic to noise ratio, long-term average spectra |
| Other measurements | Computed tomography (CT scans), magnetic resonance imaging (MRI) of the larynx |

Measurement of outcomes following voice therapy should be governed by two main principles. The first principle is that the human voice is a complex phenomenon and that multi-dimensional measurement is essential. Multiple measurements of a number of aspects of voice provide a more comprehensive method of evaluating voice change and this is clearly preferable to the use of one technique in isolation. A combination of instrumental and perceptual measures is more valuable than either one in isolation. Enderby (1992) stated that outcome measures are too often related to only one aspect of care (or one component of the disorder) and may consequently lead to a false impression of treatment effectiveness. In almost all of the literature reviewed in the chapters of this book it is clear that this multi-dimensionality of the human voice is recognised and acknowledged through the choice of a range of voice outcome measurement techniques. The second principle is that the choice of outcome measurement should be directly matched to the stated goals of the therapy intervention. Treatment can only be said to be effective if it reaches the goals that it set out to attain. The clearer the goals, the easier it is to determine whether or not these goals have been achieved. Furthermore, the clearer the goals, the easier it is to decide on the outcome measures. The critical appraisal of the voice therapy literature in the previous chapters has shown that some authors are not specific about their treatment aims prior to intervention and hence, it is often difficult to evaluate whether the outcome measures were chosen appropriately. It does, of course, allow the authors to select the outcome measures that show a significant change after therapy and discard those that do not. This is termed a "false-positive" response. The table below lists a number of possible aims of voice therapy and the techniques that could be used to measure them.

Table 2: Possible Aims of Therapy and Techniques to Measure Them

| Treatment Aim/Goal | Treatment Efficacy Criteria | Measurement Technique |
|---|---|---|
| To restore the patient's voice to normal use and function | The patient reports normal voice use | A patient questionnaire of voice use or handicap |
| To improve the quality of sound of a patient's voice to a more acceptable level | The patient's voice sounds within normal limits by "blind" listeners | A perceptual rating of voice quality |
| To improve the patient's vocal functioning so that laryngeal structure and function are normal and future phonatory trauma is minimised | Laryngeal appearance and movement appears normal to the clinician | Flexible endoscopy and stroboscopy |
| To improve the patient's voice so that he/she may return to normal work and social functioning | The patient is able to function normally in work and social situations | A patient questionnaire of vocal participation and/or handicap |
| To improve the patient's aerodynamics to enable vocal resilience | The patient has improved aerodynamic features for voice production | Aerodynamic measures such as maximum phonation time or s/z ratio |

# Important properties of voice outcome measures

## "Objective" vs "subjective" voice outcome measures

There is still an ongoing debate regarding the relative merits of "objective" and "subjective" measures of voice. In the voice literature, the term 'objective' is often used synonymously with "instrumental" and the term "subjective" is often used synonymously with "perceptual" measures. There is a misconception that "objective" measurement in this case means "exhibiting facts uncoloured by opinions" (Collins Dictionary, 1991). 'Objective' measures of voice outcome still require significant interpretation and are therefore still susceptible to bias or opinion. Equally, subjective voice outcome measures were often perceived as unreliable and reliant upon poorly defined descriptive comment. However, it is now recognised that both types of outcome measure have a place in evaluating change over time and that careful administration and reporting can enable both instrumental and perceptual voice outcome measures to be reliable and robust.

## Reliability of a measure

Reliability refers to the consistency of a measuring instrument. Liamputtong (2014) describes reliability as "the extent to which a measurement instrument is dependable, stable and free from measurement error when repeated under identical conditions" (page 168). Determining the reliability of an outcome measure is an essential component of deciding the instrument's adequacy. It is critical to the process of determining treatment effectiveness that the investigators are confident that any changes in voice outcome cannot be due to measurement inconsistency. Equally important in this context is the consistency and precision of the protocol and administration of the outcome measurement tool. An otherwise reliable measuring instrument can be inconsistent and unstable if the protocol of measurement is administered in a variable manner (Streiner and Norman, 2008). Reliability evaluates the extent to which the scores for people who have not changed are the same for repeated measures under identical conditions. These reliability measures are commonly reported in the voice literature for perceptual measures (such as rating of voice quality). There is a strong argument that these procedures should be reported for all voice outcome measurements. Reliability measures include:

- Test-retest reliability – which examines the extent to which a stable evaluation can be obtained on two different occasions when no change has taken place
- Intra-rater reliability – which examines the extent to which the same person can rate the same performance consistently
- Inter-rater reliability – which examines the extent to which different people rate the same performance consistently.

## Validity of a measure

Validity refers to whether the measurement technique measures what it is supposed to. Liamputtong (2014) describes validity as "the degree to which a scale [or instrument] measures what it is intended to measure" (page 170). The assessment of validity is a subjective judgement and is not an "all or nothing" concept; it often requires the fathering of evidence over a period of time. The different types of validity commonly referred to in voice outcomes literature are:

- **Content validity (and face validity)**
  Content validity is the extent to which the instrument covers the features that it is intended to measure. It also refers to the exclusion of items that are not

relevant to what is being measured. This is commonly seen in questionnaire design, where irrelevant or duplicate questions are omitted from the revised version. Face validity is a form of content validity and refers to the extent to which an outcome tool appears to evaluate what it is supposed to and seems plausible by the users.

- **Construct validity**
  Construct validity refers to the extent to which an instrument measures the underlying beliefs and theories that underpin that measure. Liamputtong (2014) describes three steps in establishing construct validity: (1) explicitly describing the theoretical constructs; (2) developing an assessment that attempt to directly measure these constructs; (3) testing the relationship between the constructs and the items that have been measured using the new tool.

- **Criterion validity (including concurrent and predictive validity)**
  Criterion validity refers to the extent to which the instrument in question correlates with another criterion measure (ideally a "gold standard" test that has been widely used and accepted). If both tests are administered on the same population and at the same time (concurrently), then the correlation between the two tests should be very high and the target test is said to be a valid *predictor* of the criterion score.

## Sensitivity to change of a measure ('responsiveness')

Sensitivity to change or "responsiveness" of an outcome measure refers to the extent that the instrument is able to measure relevant and important clinical change following an intervention. Clearly a measure may be "too sensitive" and produce copious data on small irrelevant natural variations. Equally, a measure may not be sensitive enough and miss important clinical changes. This involves complex decisions using concepts such as "minimal clinically important change" and "the smallest detectable difference" (Beckerman *et al.*, 2001). These concepts are concerned with determining how much change is required for it to be considered 'important'. The reliability of an instrument is key to its likely sensitivity to change. Tools with high reliability and, therefore, low measurement error are likely to be more responsive to the feature that is being measured. There has been some valuable work in certain areas of voice outcome measurement research with respect to sensitivity to change and these studies will be discussed in the relevant sections below.

## Utility

Utility refers to how simple an instrument is for use by both the clinician and the target population group. These instruments will of course differ in different clinical settings and with different population groups. Instrument utility is commonly measured by simple metrics such as time taken to complete or time allocation in addition to usual appointment, as well as qualitative feedback from clinicians and patients.

## Voice outcome measures commonly used in the efficacy literature

The following sections of this chapter represent a summary of main voice outcome measures and how they have been used in the literature in the past 10 to 15 years. Each main voice outcome measurement technique will be described. This is followed by a summary of the voice therapy efficacy studies that have used this technique to measure change over time.

### Patient ratings of voice-related quality of life

A number of patient questionnaires focus on different aspects of voice-related quality of life. In most cases these instruments have been well developed and tested for reliability and internal validity. These include:

- The Voice Handicap Index (Jacobson *et al.*, 1997)
- The Vocal Performance Questionnaire (Carding *et al.*, 1999)
- Voice Related Quality of Life (Hogikyan *et al.*, 1999)
- Voice Activity and Participation Profile (Ma and Yiu, 2001)
- The Vocal Symptom Index (Voiss) (Deary *et al.*, 2003)
- The Voice Handicap Index-10 (Rosen *et al.*, 2004).

These questionnaires focus on different components of the patient's experience of being dysphonic. All the questionnaires produce a total severity score. Some of the instruments provide sub-scale data in addition to the overall score. Patient ratings of voice-related quality of life are considered as a highly valid aspect of voice therapy evaluation. Some of these scales have been subjected to detailed factor analysis to determine construct validity (Deary *et al.*, 2004; Wilson *et al.*, 2004). The Voice Handicap Index (Jacobson *et al.*, 1997) has also been refined to a smaller VHI -10 (Rosen *et al.*, 2004) in order to address concerns about content validity and general utility.

The table below illustrates which specific voice quality of life measurement tools have been used with each treatment outcome study from 2000–2015. The full reference to each of these studies can be found in the relevant specific chapter.

Table 1: Patient Ratings of Voice-Related Quality of Life Measures in the Literature

| Year | First Author | Title | Type of Voice Problem | Outcome Measures Used |
|---|---|---|---|---|
| 2001 | MacKenzie | Does voice therapy work? A randomised control trail of the efficacy of voice therapy for dysphonia | Functional dysphonia | VPQ |
| 2002 | Sellars | Characterisation of effective primary voice therapy for dysphonia | | VPQ |
| 2003 | Beranova | New opportunities in the treatment of dysphonia | Functional dysphonia | VRQoL |
| 2004 | van der Merwe | The voice use reduction programme | Vocal nodules | Self-designed patient experience |
| 2004 | Rattenbury | Evaluating the effectiveness and efficiency of voice therapy using transnasal flexible laryngoscopy: a randomised controlled trial | Functional dysphonia | VPQ |
| 2006 | Gillivan-Murphy | The effectiveness of a voice treatment approach for teachers with self-reported voice problems. | Functional dysphonia | VRQoL VoiSS |

| Year | First Author | Title | Type of Voice Problem | Outcome Measures Used |
|------|--------------|-------|----------------------|----------------------|
| 2006 | Simberg | The resonance tube method in voice therapy: description and practical implementations | Functional dysphonia | VRQoL |
| 2007 | Spielman | Effects of an extended version of the Lee Silverman Voice Treatment on voice and speech in Parkinson's disease | Parkinson's disease | VHI |
| 2007 | Chen | Outcome of resonant voice therapy for female teachers with voice disorders: perceptual, physiological, acoustic, aerodynamic and functional measurements | Functional dysphonia | VHI |
| 2007 | Van Lierde | Long-term outcome of hyperfunctional voice disorders based on a multi-parameter approach | Functional dysphonia | VHI |
| 2008 | Niebudek-Bogusz | Acoustic analysis with vocal loading test in occupational voice disorders: Outcomes before and after voice therapy | Vocal nodules | VHI |
| 2008 | Ilomaki | Effects of voice training and voice hygiene education on acoustic and perceptual speech parameters and self-reported wellbeing in female teachers | Functional dysphonia | VHI |
| 2008 | Schindler | Vocal improvement after voice therapy in unilateral vocal fold paralysis | Vocal fold paralysis | VHI |

| Year | First Author | Title | Type of Voice Problem | Outcome Measures Used |
|---|---|---|---|---|
| 2009 | Nguyen | Randomised controlled trial of vocal function exercises on muscle tension dysphonia in Vietnamese female teachers | Functional dysphonia | Self-designed tool |
| 2010 | Cantarella | Voice therapy for laryngeal hemiplegia: the role of timing of initiation of therapy | Vocal fold paralysis | VHI |
| 2010 | Morsomme | Subjective evaluation of the long-term efficacy of speech therapy on dysfunctional dysphonia | Functional dysphonia | VHI-10 |
| 2011 | Kleemola | Twelve-month clinical follow-up of voice patient's recovery using the VAPP | Functional dysphonia | VAPP |
| 2011 | Cho | Analysis of factors influencing voice quality and therapeutic approaches in vocal polyp patients | Vocal fold polyps | VHI |
| 2012 | Halpern | Innovative technology for the assisted delivery of intensive voice treatment (LSVT (R) LOUD) for Parkinson disease | Parkinson's disease | VHI |
| 2012 | Marszalek | Assessment of the influence of osteopathic myofascial techniques on normalisation of the vocal tract functions in patients with occupational dysphonia | Functional dysphonia | VHI |
| 2012 | McCullough | Treatment of laryngeal hyperfunction with flow phonation; a pilot study | Functional dysphonia | VHI |

| Year | First Author | Title | Type of Voice Problem | Outcome Measures Used |
|---|---|---|---|---|
| 2012 | Law | The effectiveness of group voice therapy; a group climate perspective | Functional dysphonia | VAPP |
| 2012 | Shih | Singing in groups for Parkinson's disease (SING-PD): A pilot study of group singing therapy for PD-related voice/speech disorders | Parkinson's disease | VRQOL VHI |
| 2013 | Schindler | Multi-dimensional assessment of vocal changes in benign vocal fold lesions after voice therapy | Reinke's oedema, polyps and cysts | VHI |
| 2014 | Estes | Vocal fold pseudocyst: results of 46 cases undergoing a uniform treatment algorithm | Vocal pseudocysts | VHI-10 |
| 2014 | Lin | Effect of voice training in the voice rehabilitation of patients with vocal cord polyps after surgery | Vocal fold polyps | VHI |
| 2014 | Wenke | Is more intensive better? Client and service provider outcomes for intensive versus standard therapy schedules for functional dysphonia | Functional dysphonia | VHI |
| 2014 | Watts | The effects of stretch and flow voice therapy on measures of vocal function and handicap | Functional dysphonia | VHI |
| 2015 | Busto-Crespo | Voice outcomes after voice therapy in unilateral vocal fold paralysis | Vocal fold paralysis | VHI-10 |
| 2015 | Tomlinson | Manual therapy and exercise to improve outcomes in patients with muscle tension dysphonia: a case series | Functional dysphonia | VHI |

| Year | First Author | Title | Type of Voice Problem | Outcome Measures Used |
|---|---|---|---|---|
| 2015 | Petrovic-Lazic | Acoustic and perceptual characteristics of the voice in patients with vocal polyps after surgery and voice therapy | Vocal fold polyps | VHI |
| 2016 | Fu | Long-term effects of an intensive voice treatment for vocal fold nodules | Vocal Nodules | VHI |
| 2016 | Tang | Timing of voice therapy: a primary investigation of voice outcomes for surgical benign vocal fold lesion patients | Vocal polyps, cysts and nodules | VHI |
| 2016 | Zhuge | An analysis of the effects of voice therapy on patients with early vocal fold polyps | Vocal polyps | VHI |

VRQOL = Voice Related Quality of Life, VoiSS = Voice Symptom Index, VRQoL = Voice Related Quality of Life, VAPP = Voice Activity Participation Profile, VHI = Voice Handicap Index, VPQ = Voice Performance Questionnaire.

## Expert perceptual rating of voice quality

Perceptual rating of voice quality requires a listener (usually an expert) to judge a voice sample on various parameters such as overall severity, roughness, breathiness etc. The listener rates the voice parameters using one of a number of published scales. These scales include:

- GRBAS (Hirano, 1981)
- Consensus Auditory Perceptual Evaluation – Voice (CAPE-V)
- The Vocal Profile Analysis Scheme (Laver *et al.*, 1981)
- Perceptual Voice Profile (Oates and Russell, 1998).

For many clinicians, the perception of voice quality is the most valid measure of outcome for any intervention that is aimed at improving voice quality. Gerratt and Kreiman (1993) suggest that patients and clinicians decide whether a treatment is successful largely according to whether the voice sounds better.

The table below illustrates which specific instruments of rating voice quality have been used with each treatment outcome study from 2000 to 2015. The full reference to each of these studies can be found in the relevant specific chapter.

Table 2: Perceptual Rating of Voice Quality in the Literature

| Year | First Author | Title | Type of Voice Problem | Outcome Measures Used |
|------|--------------|-------|----------------------|-----------------------|
| 1991 | McFarlane | Unilateral vocal fold paralysis; perceived vocal quality following three methods of treatment | Vocal fold paralysis | Non-published scale |
| 1999 | Kelchner | Etiology, pathophysiology, treatment choices and voice results for unilateral adductor vocal fold paralysis: a 3-year retrospective | Vocal fold paralysis | Non-published scale |
| 2000 | Ylilato | Voice characteristics, effects of voice therapy and long-term follow-up of contact granuloma patients | Vocal fold granuloma | Non-published scale |
| 2001 | Holmberg | Efficacy of a behaviorally based voice therapy protocol for vocal nodules | Vocal nodules | Stockholm Voice Evaluation Approach |
| 2001 | MacKenzie | Does voice therapy work? A randomised control trial of the efficacy of voice therapy for dysphonia | Functional dysphonia | Buffalo III Voice profile |
| 2002 | Sellars | Characterisation of effective primary voice therapy or dysphonia | Functional dysphonia | Buffalo III Voice Profile |

| Year | First Author | Title | Type of Voice Problem | Outcome Measures Used |
|---|---|---|---|---|
| 2004 | van der Merwe | The voice use reduction program | Vocal nodules | Non-published scale |
| 2004 | Rattenbury | Evaluating the effectiveness and efficiency of voice therapy using transnasal flexible laryngoscopy: a randomised controlled trial | Functional dysphonia | GRBAS |
| 2006 | Sapir | Effects of intensive voice treatment [the Lee Silverman Voice Treatment (LSVT)] on vowel articulation in dysarthric individuals with idiopathic Parkinson disease: acoustic and perceptual findings | Parkinson's disease | Non-published scale |
| 2006 | Simberg | The resonance tube method in voice therapy: description and practical implementations | Functional dysphonia | GRBAS |
| 2006 | Theodoros | Treating the speech disorder in Parkinson's disease online | Parkinson's disease | Non-published scale |
| 2007 | Chen | Outcome of resonant voice therapy for female teachers with voice disorders: perceptual, physiological, acoustic, aerodynamic and functional measurements | Functional dysphonia | Non-published scale |

| Year | First Author | Title | Type of Voice Problem | Outcome Measures Used |
|---|---|---|---|---|
| 2007 | Di Benedetto | Voice and choral singing treatment: a new approach for speech and voice disorders in Parkinson's disease | Parkinson's disease | Intonation ratings |
| 2007 | Van Lierde | Long-term outcome of hyper-functional voice disorders based on a multi-parameter approach | Functional dysphonia | Non-published scale |
| 2007 | Whitehill | Effect of intensive voice treatment on tone-language speakers with Parkinson's disease | Parkinson's disease | Non-published scale |
| 2008 | D'Altri | Role of early voice therapy in patients affected by unilateral vocal fold paralysis | Vocal fold paralysis | GRBAS |
| 2008 | Ilomaki | Effects of voice training and voice hygiene education on acoustic and perceptual speech parameters and self-reported well being in female teachers | Functional dysphonia | Non-published scale |
| 2008 | Schindler | Vocal improvement after voice therapy in unilateral vocal fold paralysis | Vocal fold paralysis | GR(i)BAS |
| 2009 | Nguyen | Randomised controlled trial of vocal function exercises on muscle tension dysphonia in Vietnamese female teachers | Functional dysphonia | Non-published scale |

| Year | First Author | Title | Type of Voice Problem | Outcome Measures Used |
|------|--------------|-------|----------------------|----------------------|
| 2009 | Di Bendetto | Voice and choral singing treatment: a new approach for speech and voice disorders in Parkinson's disease | Parkinson's disease | Self-devised scale |
| 2010 | Cantarella | Voice therapy for laryngeal hemiplegia: the role of timing of initiation of therapy | Vocal fold paralysis | GRBAS |
| 2010 | Constantinescu | Home-based speech treatment for Parkinson's disease delivered remotely: a case report | Parkinson's disease | Non-published scale |
| 2010 | Morsomme | Subjective evaluation of the long-term efficacy of speech therapy on dysfunctional dysphonia | Functional dysphonia | GRB (only) |
| 2011 | Colton | Spectral moment analysis of unilateral vocal fold paralysis | Vocal fold paralysis | Non-published scale |
| 2011 | Cho | Analysis of factors influencing voice quality and therapeutic approaches in vocal polyp patients | Vocal fold polyps | GRBAS |
| 2011 | Constaninescu | Treating disordered speech and voice in Parkinson's disease online: a randomised controlled non-inferiority trial | Parkinson's disease | Non-published scale |
| 2011 | Whitehill | Effect of LSVT on lexical tone in speakers with Parkinson's disease | Parkinson's disease | Non-published scale |

| Year | First Author | Title | Type of Voice Problem | Outcome Measures Used |
|---|---|---|---|---|
| 2012 | Halpern | Innovative Technology for the Assisted Delivery of Intensive Voice Treatment (LSVT (R) LOUD) for Parkinson disease | Parkinson's disease | Non-published scale |
| 2012 | McCullough | Treatment of laryngeal hyperfunction with flow phonation; a pilot study | Functional dysphonia | CAPE-V |
| 2013 | Schindler | Multi-dimensional assessment of vocal changes in benign vocal fold lesions after voice therapy | Reinke's oedema, polyps and cysts | GIRBAS |
| 2014 | El-Banna | Early voice therapy in patients with unilateral vocal fold paralysis | Vocal fold paralysis | GRBAS |
| 2014 | Lin | Effect of voice training in the voice rehabilitation of patients with vocal cord polyps after surgery | Vocal fold polyps | GRBAS |
| 2014 | Ogawa | Immediate effects of humming on computed electroglottographic parameters in patients with muscle tension dysphonia | Functional dysphonia | Roughness rating only |
| 2015 | Fu | Intensive versus traditional voice therapy for vocal nodules: perceptual, physiological, acoustic and aerodynamic changes | Vocal nodules | GRBAS scale |

| Year | First Author | Title | Type of Voice Problem | Outcome Measures Used |
|------|--------------|-------|----------------------|----------------------|
| 2016 | Fu | Long-term effects of an intensive voice treatment for vocal fold nodules | Vocal nodules | GRBAS scale |
| 2015 | Mathur | Efficacy of voice therapy in teachers; using a perceptual assessment protocol | Functional dysphonia | CAPE-V |
| 2015 | Petrovic-Lazic | Acoustic and perceptual characteristics of the voice in patients with vocal polyps after surgery and voice therapy | Vocal fold polyps | GRB (only) |

Table 2 illustrates a number of important points. First, despite the development of voice quality rating scales with proven reliability and validity, a number of studies chose to use a non-published scale. Second, the most commonly used published rating scale is GRBAS (Hirano, 1981). Third, a number of studies have adapted the GRABS for their specific study needs. This has involved the addition of an extra parameter (for example, for instability) or deletion of a less reliable or useful parameter (for example, "aesthenia" or "strain").

## Expert rating of laryngeal function (endoscopy/stroboscopy)

Laryngeal images (using continuous light, stroboscopy or videokymography) can be interpreted using individual visual perceptual judgements. These judgements have the same validity and reliability issues as auditory perceptual ratings (Aronson and Bless, 2009). Also, similar to auditory perceptual ratings, training experience may have a significant impact on rater reliability and rating validity (Poburka and Bless, 1998). Several attempts have been made to develop different stroboscopic rating forms (Sercarz *et al.*, 1991; Dejonckere *et al.*, 1998; Poburka, 1999; Woo, 2010). However, there remains a lack of data in the literature about the specificity and sensitivity of the stroboscopic parameters that discriminate between normal and pathological voices. One published rating scale is The Stroboscopy Evaluation Rating Form (SERF) (Poburka, 1999).

The table below illustrates which specific tools rating laryngeal function have been used in any treatment outcome study reported in this book. The full reference to each of these studies can be found in the relevant specific chapter.

Table 3: Ratings of Laryngeal Function in the Literature

| Year | First Author | Title | Type of Voice Problem | Outcome Measures Used |
|---|---|---|---|---|
| 1999 | Kelchner | Etiology, pathophysiology, treatment choices and voice results for unilateral adductor vocal fold paralysis: a 3-year retrospective | Vocal fold paralysis | Stroboscopy rating |
| 2001 | Holmberg | Efficacy of a behaviorally based voice therapy protocol for vocal nodules | Vocal nodules | Laryngoscopy ratings |
| 2003 | Holmberg | Aerodynamic and acoustic voice measurements of patients with vocal nodules: Variation in baseline and changes across voice therapy | Vocal nodules | Laryngoscopy ratings |
| 2004 | van der Merwe | The voice use reduction program | Vocal nodules | Laryngoscopy ratings |
| 2005 | Leonard | Effects of voice therapy on vocal process granuloma: a phonoscopic approach | Vocal fold granuloma | Laryngoscopy ratings |
| 2006 | Simberg | The resonance tube method in voice therapy: description and practical implementations | Functional dysphonia | Laryngoscopy ratings |

| Year | First Author | Title | Type of Voice Problem | Outcome Measures Used |
|---|---|---|---|---|
| 2007 | Chernobelsky | The treatment and results of voice therapy amongst professional classical singers with vocal fold nodules | Vocal nodules | Stroboscopy ratings |
| 2007 | Chen | Outcome of resonant voice therapy for female teachers with voice disorders: perceptual, physiological, acoustic, aerodynamic and functional measurements | Functional dysphonia | Stroboscopy ratings |
| 2003 | Khidr | Effects of the "Smith Accent Technique" of voice therapy on the laryngeal functions and voice quality of patients with unilateral vocal fold paralysis | Vocal fold paralysis | Stroboscopy ratings |
| 2008 | D'Altri | Role of early voice therapy in patients affected by unilateral vocal fold paralysis | Vocal fold paralysis | Videostroboscopy ratings |
| 2008 | Niebudek-Bogusz | Acoustic analysis with vocal loading test in occupational voice disorders: Outcomes before and after voice therapy | Vocal nodules | Laryngoscopy ratings |
| 2008 | Schindler | Vocal improvement after voice therapy in unilateral vocal fold paralysis | Vocal fold paralysis | Videostroboscopy ratings |

| Year | First Author | Title | Type of Voice Problem | Outcome Measures Used |
|------|--------------|-------|----------------------|----------------------|
| 2009 | Klein | Spontaneous resolution of hemorrhagic polyps of the true vocal fold | Vocal fold polyps | Stroboscopy ratings |
| 2010 | Cantarella | Voice therapy for laryngeal hemiplegia: the role of timing of initiation of therapy | Vocal fold paralysis | Stroboscopy ratings |
| 2011 | Cho | Analysis of factors influencing voice quality and therapeutic approaches in vocal polyp patients | Vocal fold polyps | Stroboscopy ratings |
| 2011 | Mattioli | The role of early voice therapy in the incidence of motility recovery in unilateral vocal fold paralysis | Vocal fold paralysis | Stroboscopy ratings |
| 2012 | Marszalek | Assessment of the influence of osteopathic myofascial techniques on normalisation of the vocal tract functions in patients with occupational dysphonia | Functional dysphonia | Laryngoscopy ratings |
| 2012 | Nakagawa | Resolution of vocal fold polyps with conservative treatment | Vocal fold polyps | Stroboscopy ratings |
| 2013 | Halawa | Effectiveness of laryngostroboscopy for monitoring the evolution of functional dysphonia after rehabilitator treatment | Functional dysphonia | Stroboscopy ratings |

| Year | First Author | Title | Type of Voice Problem | Outcome Measures Used |
|---|---|---|---|---|
| 2013 | Schindler | Multidimensional assessment of vocal changes in benign vocal fold lesions after voice therapy | Reinke's oedema, polyps and cysts | Stroboscopy ratings |
| 2014 | El-Banna | Early voice therapy in patients with unilateral vocal fold paralysis | Vocal fold paralysis | Stroboscopy ratings |
| 2015 | Busto-Crespo | Voice outcomes after voice therapy in unilateral vocal fold paralysis | Vocal fold paralysis | |
| 2015 | Garcia Perez | Synchronous electrical stimulation of laryngeal muscles: an alternative for enhancing recovery of unilateral recurrent laryngeal nerve paralysis | Vocal fold paralysis | Videostroboscopy ratings |
| 2015 | Mattioli | Results of early versus intermediate or delayed voice therapy in patients with unilateral vocal fold paralysis: our experience in 171 patients | Vocal fold paralysis | Videostroboscopy ratings |
| 2015 | Fu | Intensive versus traditional voice therapy for vocal nodules: perceptual, physiological, acoustic and aerodynamic changes | Vocal nodules | Stroboscopy ratings |
| 2016 | Fu | Long-term effects of an intensive voice treatment for vocal fold nodules | Vocal nodules | Stroboscopy ratings |

Table 3 shows that stroboscopic and laryngoscopic ratings are commonly used as outcome measures for organic voice disorders and vocal fold paralysis disorders. This makes perfect sense and illustrates, at least to some extent, a choice of outcome measure that is related to the intervention goal. Interestingly, expert rating of laryngeal function has not been commonly used as an outcome measure in Parkinson's disease (PD). This is despite the need to understand the complex physiology of PD voice production and despite the documented risk of developing laryngeal hyperfunction as an unwanted consequence of LSVT®. It is important to note that most studies do not describe how the laryngeal and stroboscopic images are rated (i.e., the use of a published rating scale) and there are no examples of studies that report inter-rater and intra-rater reliability in these outcome studies.

## Acoustic measures of vocal output

Measurement of features of the speech/voice waveform constitutes one of the most common measures of voice quality change in the voice treatment efficacy literature. Analysis of the sound waveform is based on the fact that laryngeal pathology alters the normal vibration of the vocal folds and that there is a relationship between the vibratory patterns at the glottal source and certain parameters of the acoustic waveform generated by this vibration. A large number of different acoustic parameters can be measured and there is a variety of different calculation methods for the same acoustic parameter (Carding *et al.*, 2009). There is no standard methodology for capturing or analysing the voice samples (Brockman *et al.*, 2011). The most common acoustic waveform analyses examine features of sustained vowel samples. The main parameters are:

- Frequency perturbation measures ("jitter")
- Amplitude perturbation measures ("shimmer")
- Long-term average spectra
- Harmonics to noise ratio
- Signal to noise ratio

The table below illustrates which specific acoustic analysis tools have been used in any treatment outcome study from 2000–2015. The full reference to each of these studies can be found in the relevant specific chapter.

## Table 4: Acoustic Analysis Outcomes in the Literature

| Year | First Author | Title | Type of Voice Problem | Outcome Measures Used |
|---|---|---|---|---|
| 2000 | Ylilato | Voice characteristics, effects of voice therapy and long-term follow-up of contact granuloma patients | Vocal fold granuloma | $F_o$ Jitter Shimmer |
| 2001 | Holmberg | Efficacy of a behaviourally based voice therapy protocol for vocal nodules | Vocal nodules | SPL $F_o$ |
| 2001 | MacKenzie | Does voice therapy work? A randomised control trial of the efficacy of voice therapy for dysphonia | Functional dysphonia | Jitter Shimmer |
| 2003 | Holmberg | Aerodynamic and acoustic voice measurements of patients with vocal nodules: Variation in baseline and changes across voice therapy | Vocal nodules | SPL $F_o$ Spectral measures |
| 2004 | van der Merwe | The voice use reduction program | Vocal nodules | Unspecified parameters |
| 2007 | Chernobelsky | The treatment and results of voice therapy amongst professional classical singers with vocal fold nodules | Vocal nodules | $F_o$ Jitter Shimmer SNR |
| 2007 | Chen | Outcome of resonant voice therapy for female teachers with voice disorders: perceptual, physiological, acoustic, aerodynamic and functional measurements | Functional dysphonia | $F_O$ measures |

| Year | First Author | Title | Type of Voice Problem | Outcome Measures Used |
|---|---|---|---|---|
| 2007 | Whitehill | Effect of intensive voice treatment on tone-language speakers with Parkinson's disease | Parkinson's disease | $F_O$ measures |
| 2007 | Van Lierde | Long-term outcome of hyperfunctional voice disorders based on a multi-parameter approach | Functional dysphonia | Dysphonia Severity Rating |
| 2008 | D'Altri | Role of early voice therapy in patients affected by unilateral vocal fold paralysis | Vocal fold paralysis | $F_O$ measures Jitter Shimmer NHR |
| 2008 | Niebudek-Bogusz | Acoustic analysis with vocal loading test in occupational voice disorders | Functional dysphonia | Mean $F_o$ Jitter Shimmer RAP PPQ APQ NHR |
| 2008 | Ilomaki | Effects of voice training and voice hygiene education on acoustic and perceptual speech parameters and self-reported well being in female teachers | Functional dysphonia | Mean $F_o$ Jitter Shimmer |
| 2008 | Niebudek-Bogusz, | The effectiveness of voice therapy for teachers with dysphonia | Functional dysphonia | Mean $F_o$ Voice intensity (SPL) $F_O$ range |
| 2008 | Schindler | Vocal improvement after voice therapy in unilateral vocal fold paralysis | Vocal fold paralysis | Jitter Shimmer NHR SNR |

| Year | First Author | Title | Type of Voice Problem | Outcome Measures Used |
|---|---|---|---|---|
| 2009 | Mathieson | Laryngeal manual therapy; a preliminary study to examine its treatment effects in the management of muscle tension dysphonia | Functional dysphonia | RAP |
| 2009 | Nguyen | Randomised controlled trial of vocal function exercises on muscle tension dysphonia in Vietnamese female teachers | Functional dysphonia | Jitter Shimmer HNR Mean $F_o$ |
| 2010 | Cantarella | Voice therapy for laryngeal hemiplegia: the role of timing of initiation of therapy | Vocal fold paralysis | Jitter Shimmer NHR SNR |
| 2010 | Van Lierde | The treatment of muscle tension dysphonia: a comparison of two treatment techniques by means of an objective multiparameter approach | Functional dysphonia | Dysphonia Severity Index |
| 2011 | Stepp | Effects of voice therapy on relative fundamental frequency during voice offset and onset in patients with vocal hyperfunction | Functional dysphonia | Relative $F_o$ |
| 2011 | Cho | Analysis of factors influencing voice quality and therapeutic approaches in vocal polyp patients | Vocal fold polyps | Jitter Shimmer NHR |
| 2011 | Colton | Spectral moment analysis of unilateral vocal fold paralysis | Vocal fold paralysis | Spectral analysis |

| Year | First Author | Title | Type of Voice Problem | Outcome Measures Used |
|---|---|---|---|---|
| 2011 | Constaninescu | Treating disordered speech and voice in Parkinson's disease online: a randomised controlled non-inferiority trial | Parkinson's disease | $F_O$ range |
| 2011 | Mattioli | Results of Early Versus Intermediate or Delayed Voice Therapy in Patients With Unilateral Vocal Fold Paralysis: Our Experience in 171 Patients | Vocal fold paralysis | Jitter Shimmer NHR |
| 2011 | Whitehill | Effect of LSVT on Lexical Tone in Speakers with Parkinson's disease | Parkinson's disease | $F_O$ measures |
| 2012 | McCullough | Treatment of laryngeal hyperfunction with flow phonation; a pilot study | Functional dysphonia | NHR |
| 2013 | Schindler | Multidimensional assessment of vocal changes in benign vocal fold lesions after voice therapy | Reinke's oedema, polyps and cysts | $F_O$ Jitter Shimmer NHR |
| 2015 | Garcia Perez | Synchronous electrical stimulation of laryngeal muscles: an alternative for enhancing recovery of unilateral recurrent laryngeal nerve paralysis | Vocal fold paralysis | $F_O$ Jitter Shimmer NHR NNE |
| 2014 | Lin | Effect of voice training in the voice rehabilitation of patients with vocal cord polyps after surgery | Vocal fold polyps | Jitter Shimmer PPQ APQ NHR |

| Year | First Author | Title | Type of Voice Problem | Outcome Measures Used |
|------|--------------|-------|----------------------|----------------------|
| 2014 | Watts | The effects of stretch and flow voice therapy on measures of vocal function and handicap | Functional dysphonia | Cepstral peak performance |
| 2015 | Busto-Crespo | Voice Outcomes after Voice Therapy in Unilateral Vocal Fold Paralysis | Vocal fold paralysis | $F_o$<br>Jitter<br>Shimmer<br>NHR |
| 2015 | Fu | Intensive versus traditional voice therapy for vocal nodules: perceptual, physiological, acoustic and aerodynamic changes | Vocal nodules | Mean $F_o$<br>Jitter<br>Shimmer<br>NHR |
| 2015 | Petrovic-Lazic | Acoustic and perceptual characteristics of the voice in patients with vocal polyps after surgery and voice therapy | Vocal fold polyps | Jitter<br>Shimmer<br>APQ<br>PPQ<br>NHR |
| 2015 | Mattioli | Results of Early Versus Intermediate or Delayed Voice Therapy in Patients With Unilateral Vocal Fold Paralysis: Our Experience in 171 Patients | Vocal fold paralysis | Jitter<br>Shimmer<br>NHR<br>NNE |
| 2015 | Sale | The Lee Silverman Voice Treatment (LSVT®) speech therapy in progressive supranuclear palsy | Parkinson's disease | $F_O$ measures |
| 2015 | Sauvageau | Impact of the LSVT on vowel articulation and coarticulation in Parkinson's disease | Parkinson's disease | Acoustic formant frequencies |

| Year | First Author | Title | Type of Voice Problem | Outcome Measures Used |
|------|--------------|-------|----------------------|----------------------|
| 2016 | Tang | Timing of Voice Therapy: A Primary Investigation of Voice Outcomes for Surgical Benign Vocal Fold Lesion Patients | Vocal polyps, cysts and nodules | Jitter Shimmer Dysphonia Severity Index NHR |
| 2016 | Zhuge | An analysis of the effects of voice therapy on patients with early vocal fold polyps | Vocal polyps | Dysphonia Severity Index |

SPL= Sound pressure level, RAP = Relative Average Perturbation, PPQ = Pitch Perturbation Quotient, APQ = Amplitude Perturbation Quotient, NHR = Noise to Harmonic Ratio, $F_O$ = Fundamental frequency.

Table 4 illustrates that there remain a large number of acoustic measures of vocal output that are employed as voice outcome measures in studies of treatment effectiveness. This is despite the lack of inter- and intra-user reliability data to support these techniques. Acoustic analysis of the sound waveform can produce a large number of indices and parameters, as evidenced in Table 4. There is a significant risk of bias in post-hoc selection of the acoustic parameters that best support the author's hypotheses. Justification for the exact choice of parameter (for example, jitter, percentage jitter, relative frequency perturbation, frequency perturbation, relative jitter) is rarely provided. To many clinicians, the sole use of acoustic analysis without additional voice outcome measurements would invalidate the study as a meaningful examination of treatment effectiveness.

## Other measures

A number of additional outcome measures have been used in the voice treatment literature. These include measurements of aerodynamic performance, electroglottography and composite dysphonic severity indices. The full reference to each of these studies can be found in the relevant specific chapter.

Table 5: Other Miscellaneous Voice Outcome Measures in the Literature

| Year | First Author | Title | Type of Voice Problem | Outcome Measures Used |
|---|---|---|---|---|
| 2001 | MacKenzie | Does voice therapy work? A randomised control trial of the efficacy of voice therapy for dysphonia | Functional dysphonia | HADS<br>SF-36 |
| 2003 | Holmberg | Aerodynamic and acoustic voice measurements of patients with vocal nodules: Variation in baseline and changes across voice therapy | Vocal nodules | Transglottal air pressure<br>AC Flow<br>EGG<br>Maximum flow declination rate |
| 2003 | Beranova | New opportunities in the treatment of dysphonia | Functional dysphonia | Phonetogram (VRP) |
| 2004 | Rattenbury | Evaluating the effectiveness and efficiency of voice therapy using transnasal flexible laryngoscopy: a randomised controlled trial | Functional dysphonia | EGG |
| 2005 | Leonard | Effects of voice therapy on vocal process granuloma: a phonoscopic approach | Vocal fold granuloma | MPT<br>Airflow rates |
| 2006 | Sapir | Effects of intensive voice treatment [the Lee Silverman Voice Treatment (LSVT)] on vowel articulation in dysarthric individuals with idiopathic Parkinson disease: acoustic and perceptual findings | Parkinson's disease | SPL<br>Spectography |

| Year | First Author | Title | Type of Voice Problem | Outcome Measures Used |
|---|---|---|---|---|
| 2006 | Theodoros | Treating the speech disorder in Parkinson's disease online | Parkinson's disease | SPL |
| 2007 | Spielman | Effects of an extended version of the Lee Silverman Voice Treatment on voice and speech in Parkinson's disease | Parkinson's disease | SPL |
| 2007 | Chernobelsky | The treatment and results of voice therapy amongst professional classical singers with vocal fold nodules | Vocal nodules | S/Z ratio |
| 2007 | Chen | Outcome of resonant voice therapy for female teachers with voice disorders: perceptual, physiological, acoustic, aerodynamic and functional measurements | Functional dysphonia | Phonation Threshold Pressure |
| 2008 | D'Altri | Role of early voice therapy in patients affected by unilateral vocal fold paralysis | Vocal fold paralysis | MPT |
| 2008 | Niebudek-Bogusz | Acoustic analysis with vocal loading test in occupational voice disorders: Outcomes before and after voice therapy | Functional dysphonia | MPT |
| 2008 | Niebudek-Bogusz, | The effectiveness of voice therapy for teachers with dysphonia | Functional dysphonia | MPT |

| Year | First Author | Title | Type of Voice Problem | Outcome Measures Used |
|---|---|---|---|---|
| 2008 | Schindler | Vocal improvement after voice therapy in unilateral vocal fold paralysis | Vocal fold paralysis | MPT |
| 2008 | Tindall | Videophone-delivered voice therapy: A comparative analysis of outcomes to traditional delivery for adults with Parkinson's disease | Parkinson's disease | SPL |
| 2007 | Di Benedetto | Voice and choral singing treatment: a new approach for speech and voice disorders in Parkinson's disease | Parkinson's disease | MPT Functional residual capacity |
| 2009 | Howell | Delivering the Lee Sileverman Voice Treatment (LSVT) by web camera: a feasibility study | Parkinson's disease | SPL |
| 2009 | Mathieson | Laryngeal manual therapy; a preliminary study to examine its treatment effects in the management of muscle tension dysphonia | Functional dysphonia | Vocal tract discomfort scale |
| 2010 | Cantarella | Voice therapy for laryngeal hemiplegia: the role of timing of initiation of therapy | Vocal fold paralysis | MPT |
| 2010 | Constantinescu | Home-based speech treatment for Parkinson's disease delivered remotely: a case report | Parkinson's disease | SPL MPT |

| Year | First Author | Title | Type of Voice Problem | Outcome Measures Used |
|------|--------------|-------|----------------------|----------------------|
| 2010 | Van Lierde | The treatment of muscle tension dysphonia: a comparison of two treatment techniques by means of an objective multi-parameter approach | Functional dysphonia | Dysphonia Severity Index |
| 2011 | Constaninescu | Treating disordered speech and voice in Parkinson's disease online: a randomised controlled non-inferiority trial | Parkinson's disease | SPL MPT |
| 2011 | Mattioli | Results of early versus intermediate or delayed voice therapy in patients with unilateral vocal fold paralysis: Our experience in 171 patients | Vocal fold paralysis | MPT $F_o$ |
| 2012 | Cannito | Sentence intelligiblity before and after voice treatment in speakers with idiopathic Parkinson's disease | Parkinson's disease | SPL |
| 2012 | Halpern | Innovative technology for the assisted delivery of intensive voice treatment (LSVT (R) LOUD) for Parkinson disease. | Parkinson's disease | SPL |

| Year | First Author | Title | Type of Voice Problem | Outcome Measures Used |
|---|---|---|---|---|
| 2012 | Marszalek | Assessment of the influence of osteopathic myofascial techniques on normalisation of the vocal tract functions in patients with occupational dysphonia | Functional dysphonia | MPT Osteopathic laryngeal rating scale |
| 2012 | McCullough | Treatment of laryngeal hyperfunction with flow phonation; a pilot study | Functional dysphonia | Airflow measures |
| 2012 | Shih | Singing in groups for Parkinson's disease (SING-PD): A pilot study of group singing therapy for PD-related voice/speech disorders | Parkinson's disease | SPL |
| 2014 | El-Banna | Early voice therapy in patients with unilateral vocal fold paralysis | Vocal fold paralysis | Dysphonia Symptom Index |
| 2014 | Lin | Effect of voice training in the voice rehabilitation of patients with vocal cord polyps after surgery | Vocal fold polyps | MPT |
| 2014 | Watts | The effects of stretch and flow voice therapy on measures of vocal function and handicap | Functional dysphonia | s/z ratio MPT |

| Year | First Author | Title | Type of Voice Problem | Outcome Measures Used |
|---|---|---|---|---|
| 2014 | Wenke | Is more intensive better? Client and service provider outcomes for intensive versus standard therapy schedules for functional dysphonia | Functional dysphonia | AusTOMS |
| 2014 | Ogawa | Immediate effects of humming on computed electroglottographic parameters in patients with muscle tension dysphonia | Functional dysphonia | EGG |
| 2015 | Busto-Crespo | Voice outcomes after voice therapy in unilateral vocal fold paralysis | Vocal fold paralysis | MPT |
| 2015 | Fu | Intensive versus traditional voice therapy for vocal nodules: perceptual, physiological, acoustic and aerodynamic changes | Vocal nodules | MPT Mean airflow Subglottic pressure |
| 2015 | Fu | Delivery of intensive voice therapy for vocal fold nodules via telepractice: A pilot feasibility and efficacy study | Vocal nodules | MPT Mean airflow rate Subglottic pressure |
| 2015 | Garcia Perez | Synchronous electrical stimulation of laryngeal muscles: an alternative for enhancing recovery of unilateral recurrent laryngeal nerve paralysis | Vocal fold paralysis | MPT |

| Year | First Author | Title | Type of Voice Problem | Outcome Measures Used |
|---|---|---|---|---|
| 2015 | Mathur | Efficacy of voice therapy in teachers; using a perceptual assessment protocol | Functional dysphonia | S/Z ratio MPT |
| 2015 | Mattioli | Results of early versus intermediate or delayed voice therapy in patients with unilateral vocal fold paralysis: Our experience in 171 patients | Vocal fold paralysis | MPT |
| 2015 | Sale | The Lee Silverman Voice Treatment (LSVT®) speech therapy in progressive supranuclear palsy | Parkinson's disease | MPT |
| 2015 | Sauvageau | Impact of the LSVT on vowel articulation and coarticulation in Parkinson's disease | Parkinson's disease | SPL |
| 2015 | Tomlinson | Manual therapy and exercise to improve outcomes in patients with muscle tension dysphonia: a case series | Functional dysphonia | Measures of cervical and jaw range of motion |
| 2015 | Guzman | Do different semi-occluded voice exercises affect vocal fold adduction differently in subjects diagnosed with hyperfunctional dysphonia? | Functional dysphonia | EGG |

EGG = Electroglottography, MPT = Maximum Phonation Time, Aus TOMS = Australian Therapy Outcome Measures, HADS = Hospital Anxiety and Depression Scale, SF36 = Short Form Health Survey 36, VRP = Voice Range Profile, SPL= Sound Pressure Level.

It is clear from this chapter that the science of voice outcome measurement is limited by a lack of consistent approach. There have been a number of positive developments over the past 20 years. For example, it is clear that unidimensional voice outcome measurements rarely exist in the recent literature. There is also perhaps less reliance on acoustic analysis and an awareness that these data require significant interpretation (and hence are not truly "objective"). More valid measures such as ratings of voice quality and patient-report ratings of voice-related quality of life are now supported by strong reliability data.

## References

*The references of individual effectiveness studies that are listed in the tables of this chapter are to be found with each relevant chapter.*

Aronson A and Bless D (2009) *Clinical Voice Disorders* New York, NY: Thieme

Beckerman H, Roebroeck ME, Lankhorst GJ et al. (2001) Smallest real difference, a link between reproducibility and responsiveness. *Quality of Life Research* 10(7):571–8

Brockmann M, Drinnan MJ, Storck C, Carding PN (2011) Reliable jitter and shimmer measurements in voice clinics: the relevance of vowel, gender, vocal intensity and fundamental frequency effects in a typical clinical task. *Journal of Voice* 25(1): 44–53

Carding P, Docherty G and Horsely I (1999) A study of the effectiveness of voice therapy in the treatment of 45 patients with non-organic dysphonia *Journal of Voice* 13: 72–104

Carding PN, Wilson JA, MacKenzie K, Deary IJ (2009) Measuring voice outcomes: state of the science review *Journal of Laryngology and Otology* 123(8): 823–9

Deary IJ, Wilson JA, Carding PN et al. (2003) VoiSS: a patient derived voice symptom scale. *Journal of Psychosomatic Research.* 54: 483–89

Deary IJ, Webb A, Mackenzie K et al. (2004) Short, self-report voice symptom scales: psychometric characteristics of the voice handicap index-10 and the vocal performance questionnaire *Otolaryngology-Head and Neck Surgery* 131(3): 232–5

Dejonckere PH, Crevier L, Elbaz E et al. (1998) Quantitative rating of video-laryngostroboscopy: a reliability study. *Revue de laryngologie - otologie - rhinologie* 119: 259–60

Enderby P (1992) Outcome measures in speech therapy; impairment, disability handicap and distress. *Health Trends* 24: 61–63

Hirano M (1981) *Clinical Examination of Voice* New York, NY: Springer-Verlag

Hogikyan ND and Sethuraman G (1999) Validation of an instrument to measure voice-related quality of life (V-RQOL). *Journal of Voice* 13(4): 557–69

Jacobson BH, Johnson A, Grywalski S et al. (1997) The Voice Handicap Index; development and validation. *American Journal of Speech and Language Pathology* 6: 66–70 doi 1044/1058-0360.0603.66

Kempster GB, Gerratt BR, Verdolini Abbott K *et al.* (2009) Consensus auditory-perceptual evaluation of voice: development of a standardized clinical protocol *American Journal of Speech-Language Pathology* **18**: 124–132. doi:10.1044/1058-0360(2008/08-0017)

Laver J, Wirz S, MacKenzie J, Hiller S (1981) The perceptual protocol for the analysis of vocal profiles: work in progress. Department of Linguistics, Edinburgh University **14**: 139–55

Liamputtong P (2014) *Research Methods in Health* Oxford: Oxford University Press

Ma E, Yiu E (2001) Voice activity and participation profile: assessing the impact of voice disorders on daily activities *Journal of Speech and Hearing Research* **44**: 511–24

Oates J, Russell A (1998) Learning voice analysis using an interactive multi-media package: development and preliminary evaluation *Journal of Voice* **12**: 500–12

Olswang LB (1998) Treatment efficacy research In: Frattali CM, *Measuring Outcomes in Speech –Language Pathology* (chapter 6) New York, NY: Thieme

Rosen CA, Lee AS, Osborne J *et al.* (2004) Development and validation of the voice handicap index-10 *Laryngoscope* **114**(9):1549–56

Poburka BJ (1999) A new stroboscopy rating form. *Journal of Voice* **13**: 403–13

Poburka BJ, Bless D (1998) A multi-media computer-based method for stroboscopy rating training *Journal of Voice* **12**: 513–26

Sercarz JA, Berke GS, Arnstein D *et al.* (1991) A new technique for quantitative measurement of laryngeal videostroboscopic images. *Archives of Otolaryngology-Head and Neck Surgery* **117**: 871–75

Streiner Dl and Norman CR (2008) *Health Measurement Scales; A Practical Guide to their Development and Use* Oxford: Oxford University Press

Wilson JA, Webb A, Carding PN *et al.* (2004) The Voice Symptom Scale (VoiSS) and the Vocal Handicap Index (VHI): a comparison of structure and content *Clinical Otolaryngology and Allied Sciences* **29**(2): 169–7

Woo P (2010) *Stroboscopy* San Diego, CA: Plural Publishing, Inc., page 350

# 9

# The future

## Paul Carding

## Introduction

For some people, the establishment of high quality evidence of treatment effectiveness represents one of the major advances in health care over the past 20 years (Sackett, 1997). However, other authors have excoriated it as a development that has reduced clinical practice to "recipe book" activities for the "betterment of insurance companies" (Mullen and Streiner, 2004). The reality probably lies somewhere in the middle. This chapter contains a debate about whether we really have achieved a major advance in speech pathology healthcare for voice disorders or whether we have just begun the long journey. This chapter will also include a discussion about whether the published studies have ironically resulted in a "cookbook approach" to therapy and a consequent de-skilling of otherwise resourceful and eclectic voice clinicians.

Do the studies presented in this book constitute an "evidence base" for speech pathology intervention in voice disorders? According to Mullen and Streiner (2004), for an area of clinical practice to be considered to have a robust evidence base, four selection criteria should be met:

(1) The treatment practices have been standardised through manuals or guidelines
(2) The treatment practices have been evaluated with controlled research designs
(3) Important outcomes have been demonstrated through the use of objective measures
(4) The research was conducted by different research teams.

These criteria perhaps need a little modification for the field of speech pathology treatment of voice disorders. It may be more appropriate to state that the four selection criteria to be met should be:

(1) The treatment practices are clearly described and readily replicated
(2) The treatment practices have been evaluated with controlled research designs
(3) Important outcomes have been demonstrated through the use of high quality outcome measures which have high validity and reliability
(4) The research findings have been confirmed by different research teams.

Accordingly, we can say that the studies described in this book constitute a healthy evidence base for speech pathology treatment of a number of voice disorders. However, the evidence is far from complete and, in some areas, of poor quality. The future of treatment effectiveness research for voice disorders may be judged on how well these new challenges are met over the next decade.

## Are there enough high quality studies?

A question that arises is whether there are enough high quality treatment effectiveness studies to enable clinicians and service providers to make evidence-based decisions on the delivery and provision of voice therapy services. Surprisingly, the evidence-base movement which places such a high premium on research has barely examined what "enough" might look like (Mullen and Streiner, 2004). No studies have looked at clinical decision-making by the speech pathologist working with voice-disordered patients and whether these decisions have been based on the available evidence or indeed, whether the evidence was appropriate to the specific needs of the case at hand. Studies into the use of evidence for medical in-patients (Ellis *et al.*, 1995) and psychiatric in-patients (Geddes *et al.*, 1996) concluded that only 53–65% of patient management was supported by high quality treatment effectiveness data. Moreover, in the case of clinicians treating medical in-patients, there was unanimous agreement that non-experimental "evidence" had strongly influenced their management decisions (Ellis *et al.*, 1995). It may be reasonable to surmise that many decisions are still made by voice clinicians which are not based on the treatment literature. Professionals should remember that when decisions are taken where little or no evidence exists, then they should do so with caution and responsibility and perhaps be even more vigilant about documenting treatment goals, describing therapy interventions and monitoring treatment outcomes.

## Evidence-based practice and individualised treatment

There is a major problem with all prospective group studies of treatment effectiveness, however well designed and executed they are. In almost all cases, the results are analysed by comparing the mean score of the experimental group with that of the control group. The problem is that reporting and analysis of means should always acknowledge individual variation around the means (the standard deviation). There is also a significant likelihood that the two groups will overlap in the distribution of the scores. While this is inevitable, it is nevertheless the case that some people in the experimental group may actually do less well in treatment than some of those in the control group who may not have receive any treatment at all. Equally, some people in the comparison group may improve more than some people in the active treatment group (Mullen and Streiner, 2004).

Whilst statistical analysis takes all of this into account, the implications of these facts are commonly overlooked. It means that even a well-researched treatment modality with 'proven' effectiveness is not going to be the correct choice for every patient. The implication is that clinicians cannot automatically apply an effective treatment technique and assume that all individuals will benefit (Seeman, 2001). This has led some critics to reject group studies as a means of determining treatment effectiveness, especially for complex interventions such as speech pathology (Pring, 1986; Reilly *et al.*, 2004; Pring 2005). Some adversaries have also been led to claim that the over-emphasis on prospective group studies (and RCTs in particular) has disenfranchised the clinician from considering the individual, which in turn has denigrated professional expertise (Mullen and Streiner, 2004). This issue is discussed in more detail below.

It is important to remember, however, that the application of knowledge of treatment effectiveness and the accepted definition of evidence-based practice has always acknowledged that the treatment choice should be highly individualised and made with expert practitioner discretion.

Statistical analysis of the data from a well-conducted prospective group study should also be able to determine the probability of how an individual with the same disorder will respond to the described treatment procedure. This value is called the 'number needed to treat' (Gigerenzer *et al.*, 2007). This is the number of people who must be treated in order for there to be one additional success. There are other similar valuable parameters which include "number needed to harm" and "number needed to screen" (Greenhalgh *et al.*, 2014) These simple additions would be most welcome in all treatment effectiveness studies in the future. It would also serve as a crucial reminder to clinicians who read the study that they cannot "blindly" apply the treatment and always expect the desired outcome. Furthermore, Greenhalgh *et al.* (2014) suggest that research findings "should be expressed in ways that most people will understand" (page 3) so that appropriate clinical decisions can be made that may not match what the "best" (average) evidence seems to suggest.

## More problems with efficacy research

It is important to appreciate what a well conducted study of intervention efficacy does not tell us. An RCT finding that a voice therapy treatment is effective for a particular disorder supports the conclusion that the treated subjects in the study experienced a relatively greater therapeutic effect than the control group subjects. These results do not elucidate the really important question of *"why?"* Why was the intervention effective or not effective? Or why was it effective for some subjects and not for others? Arguably, this depth of research would truly inform clinical practice and enable modification of intervention delivery to maximise its usefulness. Furthermore, it may lead to a greater adoption of evidence-based practice by treating clinicians and prevent injudicious, impersonal and manual approaches to therapeutic intervention.

It is clear that a major problem with efficacy research is that it has inevitably been conducted in an unrealistic and unrepresentative setting. This is no more apparent than in the researcher's attempt to control the major independent variable of subject/patient characteristics. This is most commonly achieved by specifying inclusion and exclusion criteria for participants in the study. Most patients are not so simple and many do not have a single condition which can be applied cleanly to the inclusion and exclusion criteria of patients in a research study. Applying the evidence base to patients with multiple morbidity remains problematic. Moreover, as Greenhalgh *et al.*, (2014) state "multi-morbidity affects every person differently" and hence, the skill of the informed clinician is required to apply judicious use of the evidence base.

## The next phases of research

Chapter 2 described the five-phase model of a "standard protocol" for research on the efficacy of clinical interventions (Robey, 2004). In this book we have identified that there are some areas of speech therapy practice that appear to have established a Phase 3 (Robey, 2004) and Level 1 or 2 (Joanna Briggs Institute) evidence base (Functional Dysphonia and Voice Disorders in

Parkinson's Disease). In these areas there is now a clear need to extend the evidence of treatment efficacy to real clinical situations (treatment effectiveness). As discussed in Chapter 2, Robey (2004) describes Phase 4 of the treatment efficacy/effectiveness continuum as follows:

| Phase 4 | • Using large scale effectiveness studies to determine whether the treatment effects observed in efficacy studies also translate into a clinical environment<br>• Aiming, where possible, to expand the applicability of the treatment protocol beyond stringent methodological conditions<br>• Refinement (expansion or reduction) of patient selection criteria<br>• Variations in treatment delivery, dosage and additional outcome measures<br>• Concerned with external study validity |
|---|---|

No areas of voice therapy effectiveness research have truly considered the fiscal and societal costs of having a voice disorder or treating a voice disorder. Articulating and examining the health economic aspects of voice disorders remains one of the greatest challenges for our field in the next decade. This represents Phase 5 of Robey's (2004) continuum:

| Phase 5 | • Aiming to determine the cost-effectiveness of the treatment and to assess consumer satisfaction and broader issues pertaining to the social and political environment of health service delivery<br>• Costs and values are assessed in fiscal terms through cost-effectiveness studies<br>• Costs and values are assessed in societal terms through cost-benefit analysis |
|---|---|

Some chapters in this book have identified areas of voice pathology where a majority of evidence remains at Phase 1 (Robey, 2004). Phase 1 is described as follows:

| Phase 1 | Aims to detect the presence of a therapeutic effect by using small group, case series or single case studies. Detection of an effect would provide justification for further investigation |
|---|---|

However, it is possible that this phase (and several subsequent phases) may be ignored in the clamour to publish large group trials (Pring, 2005). It is important to remember that clinicians should view every patient as an "$n = 1$"study (Mullen and Streiner, 2004). Consequently, the use of study designs such as multiple baseline assessments, ABA designs and before–after case series, combined with highly valid and reliable outcome measurement, can contribute vital research evidence which can be more widely tested in a group study design. The challenge is how to secure publication of these vital preliminary datasets.

## The danger of "recipe book" voice therapy

An over-zealous application of the principles of evidence base could result in a recipe-like, manualised approach to clinical practice at the expense of professional judgement and skill. Ironically, an evidence base could, if applied incorrectly, denigrate professional expertise. As discussed above, the undiscerning clinician could use a treatment which has proven value and conclude that the patient is to blame for limited improvement. This is perhaps more of a danger for inexperienced clinicians or those who do not have access to more senior clinicians who can help contextualise the evidence around the needs, characteristics and subtleties of any individual case. It is crucial that we remember that it is the professional who is the person who "must determine whether the evidence in the literature is applicable to a particular individual bearing in mind unique circumstances, history and the like" (Mullen and Streiner, 2004).

Mullen and Streiner (2004) describe the possibility that an over-reliance on the strictest interpretation of the evidence may result in clinical nihilism. As described above, there is a difference between evidence of treatment efficacy and application of these programmes to the real world. Hence, it is quite easy to find flaws in even the best studies and easy to justify a lack of adaptation to clinical practice. Critical appraisal of the literature can too readily become nihilistic, creating the feeling that no study can be believed and that no relevant evidence exists. The answer of course lies in the clinician being professional, balanced and informed. There is a huge difference between study limitations and fatal flaws (Mullen and Streiner, 2004). The experienced clinician is required to judge whether there are study design and implementation problems which jeopardise and invalidate the results, or whether interpretation should proceed with caution and realism.

## Is a broader view of research evidence required?

Greenhalgh *et al.* (2014) provide a vision of the evidence-base movement of the future. The authors describe a research agenda that is "much broader than critical appraisal and draws on a wider range of underpinning disciplines" (page 5). For example, evidence of the patients' experience of their illness and of their treatment would be of significant value. Similarly, analysis of the individual patient's support structures (personal, emotional, financial) and how these impact on treatment effectiveness would be an important area of research. Equally, studies of how societal attitudes and institutional policy (for the clinician and for the client) impact on treatment effectiveness will enable a clearer understanding of these variables. Acknowledgement that these individual and societal contexts are relevant to clinical outcome allows a much broader perspective of what it means to provide best-evidence healthcare. In many areas this may require qualitative research approaches. It is not clear yet how these emerging evidence bases will complement the qualitative approaches that dominate at present.

There is also a need to address the ever expanding volume of evidence that is available for a clinician in any field of practice. The success of the evidence-based movement has, ironically, caused a problem with the sheer volume of evidence available. We need to balance the need for highly detailed and complex systematic reviews with pragmatic clinician-friendly reviews. We also need to consider reporting our evidence in more user-friendly and accessible ways for both practising clinicians and patients. There is the need for publishers to present the evidence in ways that inform individualised conversations. Greenhalgh *et al.* (2014) suggest the development of "decision aids" that help clinicians and patients to "raise and answer questions about the quality and completeness of evidence" (page 5) and jointly understand and individualise the information to formulate relevant and specific therapy goals. Other suggestions include plain language summaries, flow charts and option grids (Gigerenzer *et al.*, 2007). Furthermore, we need to find ways of legitimately publishing negative (or potentially harmful) results which are equally if not more, important than reporting positive effects of intervention.

However, perhaps the most pressing need is for a greater understanding of how, why and where good quality does or does not translate into clinical practice. It is not clear how clinicians and patients find, interpret and evaluate the evidence and how this is translated into clinical decision making. It is possible to view this translation issue from the perspective of those who conduct the research and/or those who use the evidence-based information in practice (Titler *et al.*, 2001; Titler, 2008).

From the 'research conductor's' perspective there are three major steps of knowledge transfer (Nieva *et al.*, 2005) which are listed in Table 1 below.

Table 1: Three Steps of Knowledge Transfer (Nieva et al., 2005)

| Knowledge creation and distillation | • Conducting high quality research<br>• Publishing high quality research<br>• Packaging relevant research findings into "products" such as guidelines and websites |
|---|---|
| Diffusion and dissemination | • Partnering with professional "opinion leaders"<br>• Partnering with healthcare organisations<br>• Partnering with "knowledge brokers"<br>• Mass communication and targeted dissemination |
| Adoption, implementation and institutionalisation | • Facilitating organisational ownership<br>• Individual and team "piloting" change to practice<br>• Multi-disciplinary implementation<br>• Continued data collection and review (with relevance to clinical team) |

However, the stages described in Table 1 provide a less useful strategy if one considers evidence-based translation from the perspective of "users of research". Titler (2008) describes the steps of evidence-based practice from the standpoint of the clinician and/or organisation delivering the healthcare.

This book began by asking whether we still need evidence of treatment effectiveness. It is clear that for voice disorders there are some strong and robust areas and some others that are at a less developed and preliminary stage. There is very little evidence of treatment effectiveness in the real world and very little knowledge about a number of variables that could prove to be critical. Even with our "best" research we have only attempted to control for the variables that we *think* are key: patient inclusion/exclusion, treatment content and outcome measurement. It is feasible that very different variables may be equally if not more influential on treatment outcome. These variables may include patient motivation, patient family support, clinician confidence and rapport, patient resilience and life experiences of coping and the patient's diagnostic journey. Most importantly, our understanding of how to apply the evidence that we do have to individual cases and with due consideration to individual and organisational differences, remains in its infancy. This is not a problem for voice therapy or voice disorders alone; it is the next big challenge to the evidence-based practice movement.

Table 2: Steps of Knowledge Transfer for the Clinician or Organisation (Titler, 2008)

| The clinician | The organisation |
| --- | --- |
| Select a disorder or intervention | Select an area for improving health care |
| Ensure that it is relevant to a specific patient | Determine the priority for the topic to the organisation |
| Liaise with other experts/clinicians as appropriate | Formulate an EBP team of key stakeholders |
| Identify, appraise and summarise the evidence | Identify, appraise and summarise the evidence |
| Stating EBP recommendations with strength and type of evidence to support | Stating EBP recommendations with strength and type of evidence to support |
| Determine if the evidence findings are appropriate for use in practice | Determine if the evidence findings are appropriate for use in practice |
| Writing an evidence-based treatment plan | Writing an evidence-based standard specific to the organisation |
| Implement the change of therapeutic approach | Piloting the change in practice |
| Evaluate relevance, outcomes and applicability to the patient | Evaluate implementation and impact for the organisation |

# References

Ellis J, Mulligan I, Rowe J and Sackett DL (1995) Inpatient general medicine is evidence based *Lancet* 346: 407–10.

Geddes JR, Game D, Jenkins NE and Sackett DL. What proportion of psychiatrics interventions are based on randomised evidence? Quality in Health Care 1996; 5: 215–17.

Gigerenzer G, Gaissmaier W, Kurz-Milcke E *et al.* (2007) Helping doctors and patients make sense of health statistics *Psychological Science in the Public Interest* 8: 53–96.

Greenhalgh T, Howicj J and Maskrey N (2014) Evidence based medicine; a movement in crisis? British Medical Journal 348:1–7.

Mullen EJ and Streiner DL (2004) The evidence for and against evidence-based practice. *Brief Treatment and Crisis Intervention* 4(2): 111–21.

Nieva V, Murphy R, Ridley N *et al.* (2005) Advances in patient safety; from research to implementation. In: Agency for Healthcare Research and Quality *From Science to Service; A Framework for the Transfer Patient Safety in Practice* Rockville, MD: Agency for Healthcare Research and Quality.

Pring T (2005) *Research Methods in Communication Disorders* London: Whurr Publishers.

Pring TR (1986) Evaluating the effects of speech therapy for aphasics: Developing the single case methodology *International Journal of Language and Communication Disorders* **21**(1): 103–15. Article first published online: 24 Mar 2011. DOI: 10.3109/13682828609018547.

Reilly S, Douglas J, Oates J (2004) *Evidence-based Practice in Speech Pathology* London: Whurr Publishers.

Robey RR (2004) A five-phase model for clinical outcome research *Journal of Communication Disorders* **37**: 401–11.

Sackett DL, Richardson WS, Rosenberg W and Haynes RB (1997) *Evidence-based Medicine: How to Practice and Teach EBM* New York, NY: Churchill Livingstone.

Seeman MV (2001) Clinical trials in psychiatry: Do results apply to practice? *Canadian Journal of Psychiatry* **46**: 352–55.

Titler MG (2008) The evidence for evidence-based practice implementation. In: RG Hughes (Ed.) *Patient Safety and Quality: An Evidence-Based Handbook for Nurses* Rockville, MD: Agency for Healthcare Research and Quality (US), Chapter 7.

Titler MG, Klieber C, Steelman VJ *et al.* (2001) The Iowa model of evidence-based practice to promote quality care. *Critical Care Nursing Clinics of North America* **13**(4): 497–509.

# Index

Accent Method, 36, 43, 86, 90, 102, 104, 106–7
acoustic analysis, 30, 39–40, 61–2, 70, 84, 116, 136, 143, 154, 157–9, 163, 165, 171
acoustic measures, 35, 58–63, 67, 84–86, 88–91, 143, 157–8, 163–5
  amplitude perturbation measures (shimmer), 32–34, 39, 60, 63–5 69–70, 72, 86–8, 92–4, 102–4, 118, 157–63
  frequency perturbation measures (jitter), 32–4, 39, 60, 63–5, 69–70, 72, 85–8, 92–4, 102–4, 118, 157–63
  harmonics to noise ratio, 34, 85–7
  long term average spectra, 34, 65, 66, 136, 150, 157
  signal to noise ratio, 60, 63, 72, 136, 157
adherence, 57, 76–7
aerodynamic measurements. *see* measurement - aerodynamic
attendance, 67, 76–7
auditory perceptual measurements, 40, 60, 74, 76, 85, 118, 136, 146, 152
average score. *see* scores
axonotmesis, 99

bias, 3–4, 7–11, 16, 19–21, 95, 123, 125, 138, 163
breathing, 32, 35, 43, 69, 73–74, 84, 86–90, 100, 104, 115, 117, 120, 146

CAFET. *see* Computer-Aided Fluency Establishment Trainer
CAPE-V. *see* Consensus Auditory Perceptual Evaluation - Voice

case
  case series, 4, 9, 12, 15, 24, 35–7, 45, 57, 66, 88, 90, 92, 94–5, 102–3, 105, 108, 118–9, 145, 170, 177
  case studies, 4–5, 9, 12, 14, 24, 57, 62, 66, 95, 120, 125, 127, 177
  case-control study, 9, 11, 14
chance, 19, 23–4
clandestine controls, 16
clinical significance, 23
cohort study, 4–5, 9, 11, 66, 89, 92–4, 114, 124, 128
comparative study, 4, 9, 10–12, 20, 36, 41, 56, 105
Computer-Aided Fluency Establishment Trainer (CAFET), 73
confounded outcomes, 16, 19
confounding factors, 21, 91, 114
construct validity. *see* validity
consumer satisfaction, 14, 66, 177
content validity. *see* validity
control group, 4, 9, 11–12, 14, 16, 20–1, 37, 43, 64, 66, 69, 83, 87–8, 93, 105, 124, 175–6
correlation, 16, 25, 32, 41, 69, 88, 115, 140
cost effectiveness, 14, 47, 57, 177,
counselling, 35, 43, 59, 66, 85, 87
criterion validity. *see* validity
cysts, 81–5, 89, 92–4, 145–6, 151, 156, 161, 163

DBS. *see* deep brain stimulation
deep brain stimulation (DBS), 114
direct therapy, 42–4, 64, 94, 106, 108

Dopamine, 113–4, 125
dysphonia
    functional dysphonia, 27–30, 35–40, 42–7, 64, 69, 71, 142–5, 147–55, 158–62, 164–70, 176
    hyperfunctional, 27–8, 36–7, 41, 45, 55, 68–9, 72, 82–3, 90, 128, 143–4, 151, 157, 159–61, 168, 170
    muscle tension, 27–8, 35–7, 41–2, 46, 64, 69, 83, 86, 144–5, 149, 151, 160, 166–7, 169–70
    non-organic, 27–8
    psychogenic, 27, 30

EBP. *see* evidence-based practice
efficacy. *see* treatment
electromyography, 41, 100, 136
electroglottography, 34, 41, 65, 67, 163, 170
eligibility, 9, 10, 123
EMG. *see* electromyography
endoscopy *(see* also stroboscopy) 33, 59, 91, 100, 136, 138, 152
exclusion criteria, 8, 12, 14, 16–7, 21, 101, 105, 123, 176, 180
expert opinion, 3

face validity. *see* validity
Five-phase model of efficacy/effectiveness research (The), 13–4, 22, 62, 176
flow phonation therapy, 31, 35–7, 43 144, 151, 161, 168
follow-up, 30–1, 46, 57, 65, 71, 73, 90, 96, 109, 124, 144, 147, 158
functional voice disorders, *see* dysphonia - functional dysphonia
fundamental frequency, 32, 34, 41, 65, 88, 90, 104, 119–20, 125, 136, 160, 163, 171

¹ottal closure, 39, 63, 106
    setting, 13, 15, 28, 72, 91, 127, 137, 174, 179

granuloma, 81–2, 90–2, 147, 153, 158, 164

harmonic to noise ratio 34, 85–6, 88, 94, 104, 136, 157, 163
Hawthorne effect, 21
hierarchies of evidence, 4, 8–9
humming exercises, 31, 37, 41, 106, 151, 169
hypotheses, 15, 163

inclusion criteria, 9, 89, 101
indirect therapy, 42–4, 64, 94
integrity, 1–2, 17
intensity, 17, 34, 38, 40, 44–5, 58–65, 69–70, 72, 74–5, 92–4, 102–4, 107, 109, 136, 159, 171
inter-rater reliability. *see* reliability measures
interrupted time-series, 4–5, 9, 11–12
intervention effectiveness, xvii, 4–5, 8–9, 37
intra-rater reliability. *see* reliability measures

jitter. *see* acoustic measures

large-scale effectiveness studies, 14, 47, 177
laryngeal examination, 18, 39, 62, 90, 128
laryngeal microsurgery, 56
laryngeal palpation therapies. *see* manual therapies
laryngeal tension, 84, 89
laryngography, 34, 136
Lee Silverman Voice Treatment (LSVT), 117–29, 144, 148, 150–1, 157, 161–2, 164, 166–7, 170
lesions. *see* vocal fold lesions
Literature review 9, 15, 19, 137, 100, 116, 137, 178
LSVT®. *see* Lee Silverman Voice Treatment

manual therapies, 30–32, 35–6, 41, 43, 145, 160, 166, 170
mean score. *see* scores
measurement, 6, 19, 38, 72, 74, 91, 163–5
  aerodynamic, 61–64, 67, 87, 136, 138, 143, 148, 151, 153–4, 156, 158, 162–5, 169
  bias and reliability, 8, 14, 20, 139, 140, 142–3
  instruments, 14, 41, 61, 85, 139, 153–4, 158
  tools, 20, 136, 138
  outcomes, 6, 19, 20, 38–40, 47, 58, 61, 95, 129, 136,–7, 139, 141, 148, 163, 171, 178, 180
meta-analysis, 10, 29
methodology, 4, 9, 37, 39, 95, 157
MPT. *see* Maximum phonation time
mucosal wave, 39, 63, 81–2
multi-dimensional evaluation, 38

neuropraxia, 99
neurotmesis, 99
nodules. *see* vocal fold nodules
non-randomised experimental trial, 4, 9, 11

OperaVOX, 40
organic voice disorders, 6, 27, 157
outcome measure. *see* measurement

palpation rating scales. *see* manual therapies
Parkinson's Disease, xiii, xvii, xviii, 6, 113–7, 119, 121–9, 143–5, 148–51, 157, 159, 161–2, 164–8, 170, 177
patient-reported symptoms, 40
PD. *see* Parkinson's Disease
perceptual evaluation, 40–1, 146
perceptual rating, 33–4, 60, 76, 80, 85, 87, 90, 102, 104, 117–8, 121, 124, 135–6, 138, 146–7, 152
perceptual voice profile, 146
phase symmetry, 39

photoglottography, 136
pitch, 34, 39, 43, 55, 58, 61, 65, 84, 87–8, 90, 94, 115, 117, 119–20, 136, 163
pitch perturbation. *see* pitch
placebo effect (the), 20, 40, 60, 73–4, 123
polyp, 37, 60, 69, 73, 81–9, 92–4, 96, 144–6, 150–2, 155–6, 160–3, 168
post-operative voice care, 83, 85
power calculations, 8, 25, 36
probability, 19, 22–4, 175
pseudocysts, 81–2, 89, 145,
pseudo-randomised controlled trial, 4, 9–10, 93–4

qualitative data, 18, 141, 179
quantitative studies, 10, 18, 72

randomised controlled trial (RCT), 4–5, 9–11, 15, 21, 29, 35, 37, 43, 45, 56, 69, 88, 117, 119–21, 123–5, 127, 142, 144, 147–50, 158, 160–61, 164, 167, 175–6
range. *see* Scores
RCT. *see* randomised controlled trial
recurrent laryngeal nerve (RLN), 99, 156, 161, 169,
refinement, 14, 177
reflux, 81–3, 86, 90–1, 95
Reinke's oedema, 37, 84–5, 93, 145, 151, 156, 161
reliability measures
  inter-rater reliability, 18, 39–41, 90, 92, 95, 139, 157
  intra-rater reliability, 18, 33, 39–41, 95, 139, 157
  test-retest reliability, 139
research questions, 7–8, 10, 18
resonance, 36–7, 44, 89, 100, 143,
RLN. *see* recurrent laryngeal nerve

samples, 16, 24–5, 29, 57, 77, 90,
schizophrenic study type, 15
scores, 24–5, 33, 41, 43, 45, 63, 65, 85, 88, 117, 127–8, 139–41, 175

semi-occluded vocal tract therapy, 32, 35–7, 43,
sensitivity to change, 29, 39, 41, 47, 140–1, 152
service provision and delivery, 1–2, 14, 42, 66, 76–7, 127, 145, 169, 174, 177
shimmer. see acoustic measures
Signal to noise ratio. see Acoustic measures
Single arm studies, 4, 9, 12, 117–8, 121–2, 125
sound pressure level (SPL), 18, 62, 116–7, 124, 127–9, 136, 158–9, 163–8, 170
SOVT. See semi-occluded vocal tract therapy
SPL. see sound pressure level
standard deviation, 24–5, 175
statistics
  statistical tests, 6, 16, 18–19, 23, 25, 30, 84, 92–3, 102, 175
  non-parametric, 23–4
  parametric, 23–4
  statistical significance, 19, 23–5, 35, 37, 39, 45, 68–70, 72, 85–6, 88–9, 93–4, 102–4, 108–9, 128
strength of treatment, 2, 17, 181
stroboscopy, 30, 39, 61, 63–5, 81–2, 84, 86, 92–3, 102–5, 128, 138, 138, 152–7
study design xvii, 4–12, 15, 17–19, 21, 70, 91, 105, 108–9, 117–22, 135, 177–8
flaws, 8, 15, 178
systematic error. see bias
systematic review, xvii, 4–5, 9–10, 19–20, 29, 38–9, 43–4, 123–4, 179

telepractice, 45, 63, 76–7, 87, 169
teletherapy. see telepractice
test-retest reliability. see reliability measures
treatment effectiveness and efficacy, 1–2, 6, 13–14, 17–18, 22, 25, 27, 29, 35, 4, 46, 57, 66–9, 76–7, 95–6, 108–9, 123–5, 138, 141–2, 144, 147, 150, 152–3, 157–8, 164, 169–70, 176–8
typical score. see scores

unilateral vocal fold paralysis, (UVFP) xviii, 6, 28, 99–101, 105–9, 143, 145, 147, 149–151, 153–6, 159–62, 165–70,
unrepresentative samples. see samples
utility, 141–2
UVFP. see unilateral vocal fold paralysis

Validity, 6, 14, 18–22, 29, 35, 39–41, 47, 77, 125, 139–42, 152, 174, 177
VAPP. see Voice Activity and Participation Profile
variables. see variance
variance, xiii, 7–8, 10–11, 13–14, 16–19, 21–3, 25, 28, 35, 37–8, 40–1, 43–7, 71, 74–5, 85, 88, 93, 95, 104–8, 114–5, 117, 120, 124, 126, 128–9, 139–40, 153, 158, 164, 175–7, 179–80
VHI. see Voice Handicap Index
VHI-10. see Voice Handicap Index
videolaryngostroboscopy. see stroboscopy
videostroboscopy. see stroboscopy
visual perceptual measurements, 60, 136, 152,
vocal fold
  lesions, xiii, 37, 55–6, 70, 81–7, 89, 91–3, 95–6, 145, 151, 156, 161
  mass, xiii, 55, 81–3, 89, 92, 95–6,
  nodules, xiii, xviii, 6, 27, 32, 37, 45, 55–64, 66–77, 81, 83, 85, 94, 142–3, 146–8, 151–4, 156, 158, 162–5, 169
vocal function exercise, 33–4, 37, 43, 69, 89, 106, 144, 149, 160
Vocal Performance Questionnaire (The), 34, 40, 64–5, 141
Vocal Profile Analysis Scheme (The), 146
Vocal Symptom Index (VOISS) (The), 33, 40, 141–2
Voice Activity and Participation Profile (VAPP), xvii, 34, 46, 141, 146

Voice Handicap Index (VHI) (The), xvii, 30–34, 40, 43, 63, 65, 84–7, 89, 93–4, 102, 104, 117, 121–2, 128, 141–6
Voice Handicap Index-10 (VHI-10) (The). *see* Vocal Handicap Index
Voice Related Quality of Life (VRQOL), 34, 45, 141–2, 146, 171

VOISS. *see* Vocal Symptom Index
VPQ. *see* Vocal Performance Questionnaire
VRQOL. *see* Voice Related Quality of Life

CPSIA information can be obtained
at www.ICGtesting.com
Printed in the USA
BVOW04s1931121116
467681BV00002B/3/P